T0296371

The Dream Drugstore

The Dream Drugstore
Chemically Altered States of Consciousness

J. Allan Hobson

A Bradford Book
The MIT Press
Cambridge, Massachusetts
London, England

First MIT Press paperback edition, 2003

This book was set in Sabon by Achorn Graphic Services, Inc., and was printed and bound in the United States of America.

Library of Congress Cataloging-in-Publication Data

Hobson, J. Allan, 1933–
  The dream drugstore : chemically altered states of consciousness / by J. Allan Hobson.
    p. cm.
  "A Bradford book."
  Includes bibliographical references and index.
  ISBN 978-0-262-08293-8 (hc. : alk. paper)—978-0-262-58220-9 (pb. : alk. paper)
    1. Altered states of consciousness—Physiological aspects. 2. Neurochemistry.

QP411.H633 2001
612.8'2—dc21

                                                                    00-050013

To my Dreamstage collaborators,

Paul Earls,
Ragnhild Karlstrom, and
Theodore Spagna

Contents

Introduction

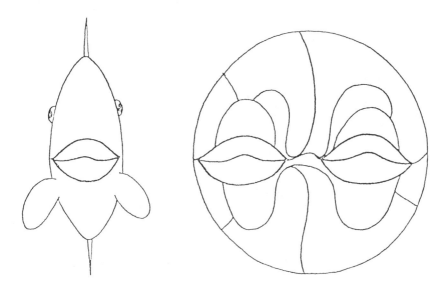

What do normal dreaming, the visions induced by psychedelic drugs, and the psychoses of mental illness have in common? One often hears the simple answer "chemical imbalance" without further explanation. But by now, we have advanced our knowledge of how the chemistry of the brain balances while we are awake and how that balance shifts when we fall asleep and dream to the point of providing the basis of a unified theory. With it, we can begin to explain, in much more specific terms, the chemical imbalances caused by psychedelic drugs, or those chemical imbalances that may cause depression and schizophrenia. From the same knowledge base we can also begin to understand how and why the drugs that doctors prescribe to correct imbalances restore the natural equilibrium of the brain.

The Dream Drugstore details the chemical balance concept in terms of what we know about the regulation of normal states of consciousness over the course of the day by the shifting balance of brain chemicals called neuromodulators. Neuromodulators have been the focus of sleep and dream research for the past 25 years. Using this knowledge as a lens through which to view the results of the psychedelic experiments of the 1960s and the descriptions of careful self observers before and since, we find striking confirmation that every drug that has potent transformative effects on consciousness interacts with the brain's own consciousness-altering chemicals.

Moreover, when we review the chemical theories of mental illness, we find further confirmation of the neuromodulatory imbalance-balance hypothesis and, in many cases, we can specify the mechanisms of pathological dysfunction in terms of what we know about normal functions. Because of the difficulties of studying human brain chemistry directly much of our theorizing is necessarily conjectural and incomplete, but the recent development of brain imaging techniques, which have revolutionized sleep and dream science, provides a strong bridge to the brain chemistry that has been detailed in animal experiments. *The Dream Drugstore* emphasizes the promise of integration across what until recently appeared to be an uncloseable gap.

In this book I develop a three-way analogy between dreaming, psychosis, and psychedelic experience. In the interest of integration, I push this analogy to the point of identity by arguing that all these conditions are altered states of consciousness caused by changes in the brain's neuromodulatory systems. As a metaphor, *The Dream Drugstore* is your chemical brain, not a building where you go to get prescriptions filled.

The first two parts of this book explain how scientists now understand normal alterations of consciousness in brain chemical terms. In part I, The Scope and Shape of Conscious States, I define the psychological components and dimensions of conscious experience. Chapter 1 shows how subjective experience can be conceptualized and measured in relation to brain science. It also introduces the notion of a unified brain-mind. Chapter 2 emphasizes the strategy of studying both spontaneous and experimental alterations in conscious state. Chapter 3 contrasts waking and dreaming by illustrating the way that we can measure these dramatic spontaneous changes in conscious state.

Modern neuroscience has permitted us to build the scientific base that Freud wanted but which psychoanalysis had to do without. Part II treats two foundational themes of psychoanalysis, dreaming (chapter 4) and dissociation (chapter 5), showing that we can understand mind, brain, and drug action within a new unified conceptual framework. To emphasize this paradigm shift, I introduce the notion of neurodynamics and show how many processes previously considered to be exclusively psychodynamic are actually embodied in brain anatomy and physiology.

Part III lays the groundwork for understanding the brain as the physical basis of consciousness. It describes the regional, cellular, and molecular mechanisms that may contribute to alterations of conscious states. Chapter 6 begins to tease apart the major subdivisions of the brain-mind and to describe their interaction in normal conscious state alteration. In chapter 7, we meet the neuromodulatory chemical systems that appear to be causative of those alterations.

To demonstrate how prone consciousness is to exaggeration, distortion, and takeover by changes in brain function, chapter 8 deals with easily understandable disorders of sleep and dreaming, and chapter 9 crosses the indistinct line separating psychiatry and neurology, considering unequivocal brain diseases that alter consciousness in dreaming and dreamlike states.

The stage is now set for three variations on the Drugstore theme.

Part IV, the Medical Drugstore, documents the ingenuity of the pharmaceutical industry in developing drugs to counteract anxiety and insomnia (chapter 10), to raise and lower mood in the treatment of depression and mania (chapter 11), and to eliminate or diminish the psychotic hallucinations and delusions of schizophrenia (chapter 12). As I praise the potency and undoubted value of many of these agents, I sound an alarm about some of the risks involved in their use by citing examples of new diseases and disorders caused by the drugs, especially with indiscriminate long-term use.

Part V, the Recreational Drugstore, talks about the good and bad trips caused by psychedelic drugs (chapter 13), the neurology of pain and narcotic analgesia (chapter 14), and then concludes with a discussion of natural drugs that made their way from ritual use to the streets, sometimes via modern pharmaceutical laboratories. This section also raises questions about the distinctions between legitimate and illegitimate drug use (chapter 15).

In part VI, the Psychological Drugstore, we come full circle back to subjectivity and consciousness itself, but now we view the mind as an agent of change, not just the vehicle or mediator of change. In this concluding section on the treatment implications of our new science I unashamedly espouse the view that the mind is de facto causal because the awareness of awareness allows us to voluntarily direct thought and hence brain activity. Besides making the mind-brain concept foundational in the reconstruction of psychology, the Psychological Drugstore specifically critiques, corrects, and updates many erroneous assumptions and practices that still impede the progress of psychoanalysis because the entire theoretical structure of psychoanalysis rests upon Freud's outmoded dream theory. *The Dream Drugstore* proposes a radical revision of dynamic psychology based upon the findings of the new neuropsychology of dreaming.

Acknowledgments

The inspiration for this book is centered on my personal experience of the 1960s and 1970s, when I saw so many friends, colleagues, and fellow Americans experiment with drugs. Drug experimentation was not something that appealed to me but I was a very curious and interested onlooker at all levels of this extraordinary cultural phenomenon.

At the same time that I was observing the effects of these drugs on people that I knew, I was investigating the neuropharmacological basis of sleep, especially REM sleep dreaming, and it occurred to me early on that there must be some common ground between these two areas of work. And that common ground is what this book is about.

In the late 1970s when rebellious drug taking was abating and sleep science was ripening, I had the impulse and the opportunity to work on an experimental theatrical piece called *Dreamstage,* which verged on the psychedelic while conspicuously avoiding drugs. In my dedication to this book, I acknowledge my collaborators in conveying to the public the deeply wondrous aesthetics of dreaming and of its scientific study.

Bringing the book to fruition was abetted by Michael Rutter's enthusiastic adoption of the proposal at MIT Press. The follow-up work of his collaborator Sara Meirowitz has been extremely helpful, especially in obtaining permission for some of the figures that illustrate a theme that I had also wanted to have be a major and prominent part of the book, namely the heroism of those self-experimenters who spoke for the many drug-takers by leaving adequate records. I particularly admire the very few who were scientifically rigorous enough to describe their experience in a way that was useful to a person like me who was interested in understanding the possible mechanisms underlying the phenomenon. One of these was my correspondent Claude Rifat, whose many informal notes to me formed an inspiration for the book and whose interesting drawings are now an integral part of this text.

In terms of the scientific database that feeds the theory, the work in the Laboratory of Neurophysiology is obviously a long-lasting, highly collaborative phenomenon. To name collaborators is always dangerous in this area because one will omit others whose role might have been as important. I mention Bob McCarley first to emphasize the early part of our work, those first sixteen years (1968–1984) when we worked together on the evolution of the reciprocal interaction and activation-synthesis models. The transition to the pharmacological tests of the model occurred just about the time that Bob was leaving the lab. People who have recently participated in that line of work are Jim Quatrocchi, Subimal Datta, and Jose Calvo. They are just three of the most recent and productive investigators in a long line going all the way back to Tom Amatruda and Tom Mackenna in the early days, and which includes Helen Baghdoyan, Ralph Lydic, Ken-Ichi Yamamoto, and Marga Rodrigo-Angulo as the validity of each of the models was established.

The work has enjoyed the unstinting support of the National Institutes of Mental Health through our grant MH 13293, lovingly administered by Izja Lederhendler; more recently our forays into cognitive science have been supported by grant MH48832 and administered by Howard Kurtzman. Our pharmacological efforts have now attracted the support of the National Institute on Drug Abuse through grant number R01 DA11744. In the development of the proposal and the pursuit of this work we are very grateful to Harold Gordon, the administrator at NIDA whose strong personal interest in sleep research and its cognitive aspects have helped us enormously.

Leadership in the cognitive science domain has been provided by Bob Stickgold, who has recently been helped in the analysis of dreaming by Roar Fosse. Ed Pace-Schott has done the lion's share of the work in the NIDA-supported projects and has provided invaluable help in the editing of this book. Any errors that remain are obviously not his responsibility, but mine.

The audacity to attempt such an integrated synthesis comes from two sources. One is Solomon Snyder's wonderful book *Drugs and the Brain*, which I reread and used frequently in writing this volume. *Drugs and the*

Brain is a daring masterpiece. It is fired by Snyder's brilliance and contains an unusual synthesis of phenomenology and basic neuroscience. Finally, the support of the MacArthur Foundation's Mind-Body Network has been important not only materially but also intellectually and spiritually. For the first time in my life, I was actually encouraged to do the sorts of experiments and indulge in the integrative modes of thinking of which I hope this book gives some adequate account.

Part I
The Scope and Shape of Conscious States

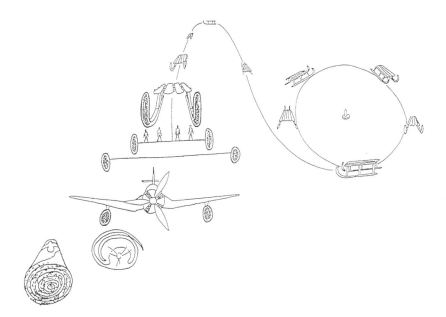

1

Consciousness and Brain Science

Normal human consciousness is so rich and so naturally variegated that any willful efforts to alter it artificially may seem, at first glance, perverse. But human beings are never satisfied with things as they are. People are always pushing the envelope of conscious experience.

Three of the reasons for our restless experimentalism are clear. In the first place, normal consciousness is *not* always pleasant. In mental illness, the impulse to alter consciousness via drugs that reduce hallucinations or elevate mood is easy to understand and to accept. Short of that, many of us feel entitled to those holidays from conscientious consciousness that a martini, a glass of wine, or a can of beer affords.

In the second place, normal consciousness can, at its natural limit, be so alluringly ecstatic as to induce a craving for more of the same. Lost elation calls for its restoration or enhancement via a stimulant booster. Such conscious state properties as creativity, sexual pleasure, and learning capacity can all be pumped up by bolstering or imitating the brain's own uppers.

In the third place, the capacity to hallucinate, to believe the impossible, and to experience visions and delusional thoughts all steeped in a broth of passionate emotion is, for normal persons as well as for the mentally ill, a variety of religious experience. At first glance it would appear that drug takers wanted to become psychotic.

But why would anyone want to cultivate the symptoms of mental illness? The answers to that question are directly related to the narrow definition of Altered States of Consciousness (ASC) that arose in the psychedelic era of the 1960s. The era's radicalism was only a recrudescence of the age-old hankering for transcendence, and it is this mystical yearning that constitutes the major motive for altering consciousness. Current reality, the superficial appearance of things, and our limited capacities to think and feel are not enough. There must be something more. We seek reality beyond appearance: the supernatural that lies above the natural world, the deity who controls our destiny, the essence of existence.

Richard Alpert's (aka Ram Dass) accounts of going from LSD to Hindu mysticism in the late 1960s is a very good example of this phenomenon. There was a resurgence of psychedelic mysticism and psychotherapy in the "New Age" movement(s) of the 1980s among people using the drug MDMA ("ecstasy"). This was an emotion-based (vs. altered perceptual) experience. The "rave" scene among young people today (also MDMA-based) is a similar, though more hedonistic, phenomenon. Whatever the motive or goal of voluntary state alteration, it is vital to understand its underlying brain mechanisms.

When I call dreaming an altered state of consciousness, I am not just being provocative. I mean to invoke and unify both naturalistic and artificial alterations of conscious state. *The Dream Drugstore* is a natural extension of a line of my work that began in *The Dreaming Brain* and *Sleep* (which were devoted to psychophysiological model building) and continued in *Dreaming as Delirium* and *Consciousness,* which broadened and deepened the model to encompass a wider range of normal and abnormal states and began to consider how exogenous chemicals might drive consciousness in one direction or another. Having earlier elaborated a brain-based model to account for the alterations of consciousness that occur naturally in dreaming, I wondered if they could help us understand the many artificial alterations of consciousness that have been induced by drugs and other interventions over the ages—but most dramatically in the last half of the twentieth century.

This book focuses on the psychopharmacology of the psychedelics and interprets their effects in terms of what we know about how the brain alters consciousness when it switches from waking to dreaming. I also apply the brain-based model of dreaming to the related phenomenon of hypnosis; these nonpharmacological altered states share the property of dissociation, for which I suggest new neurobiological underpinnings. The upshot is a brain-based alternative to the psychoanalytic paradigm of Sigmund Freud.

Psychosis, Sainthood, and Psychedelism

Seeing visions or hearing voices can only be attractive if the social context rewards and supports them and the individual believes that such experiences are valuable. Accusatory voices that arise unbidden cause fear and suspicion, leading to the belief that one is being persecuted by an external agency like the devil, Martians, or the FBI. In this case, we call the perceptions hallucinations and the beliefs delusions, and in so doing label them symptoms of mental illnesses like schizophrenia. The person with this kind of psychosis becomes a patient, with the most dire personal and social consequences.

In an earlier time, many people with visions and unprovable beliefs about their agency could become saints if their beliefs conformed to institutional rules. In the "New Age" movement(s) of the 1980s many "positive" visionaries were widely embraced as authentic and many seem still to be in more restricted circles (e.g., among movie stars). But today, even those people whose visions are beatific and confidently attributed to a benevolent God are just as likely to be called psychotic and labeled mentally ill as those who are hounded by malevolent agencies. Although they are less likely to be arrested and hospitalized against their will, their careers are usually sidetracked, their social contacts splintered, and their self-esteem badly damaged.

Whether the hallucinations and delusions that define psychosis can be voluntarily initiated and terminated is another factor determining the value attributed to psychosis. The people we call patients don't have the partial but significant volitional control that many seekers of divine communication enjoy. The wannabe saint often used voluntary deprivation of food, domestic comfort, and—most of all—sleep to set the stage for inspiring and instructive visions and messages from the Godhead. Sleep deprivation has been used in this way by religious reformers like Emanuel Swedenborg as well as by political groups bent on brainwashing. In this case, the visions, the voices, and the beliefs are not likely to be called psychotic, even though they fit the formal definition of psychosis perfectly!

Now that biochemistry has given us mind-altering pills, the modern seeker of psychosis-like transcendence has it all: voluntary control, personal meaning, and the social support of a large subculture. Psychotic experience is, in this case, the very goal of the psychedelic drug taker. Whether indulgence in recreational drugs is entirely risk free is a question that I will later consider, together with some problems associated with prescription drug-taking. The main point is that whatever the context—including dreaming—psychosis is psychosis is psychosis. To understand how psychosis can arise naturally, the best approach is to explore the physiology of normal consciousness and learn how the normal psychosis that is dreaming is engendered.

Consciousness and Its Vicissitudes

The human brain is conscious. When suitably activated, gated, and modulated, it senses, perceives, attends, feels, analyzes, acts, and remembers. Moreover, it *organizes its activities,* takes a running account of these functions in three related and highly abstract ways: first through awareness, second through a sense of a self that is aware, and third through the awareness of awareness. We now have the opportunity of finding out how all of these operations are achieved.

We can understand consciousness by applying the techniques of modern neuroscience to the study of the brain under those natural and artificial conditions that change the attributes of the brain's consciousness. The natural conditions are those related to the normal sleep-wake cycle and to its pathological vicissitudes. The artificial conditions are those behavioral and pharmacological interventions designed to alter consciousness for a wide variety of experiential and clinical purposes.

Fortunately for the scientist interested in these matters, the attributes of consciousness tend to be organized in a correlated manner, resulting in what are called states. By states we mean syndromes or clusters of attributes. When we speak of altered states of consciousness, we refer to the tendency of consciousness to be at a higher or lower level, to be concerned with external or internally generated data, and to be organized in a linear logical or parallel analogical fashion, and to be more or less affect driven.

Both the natural and artificial conditions that alter consciousness affect one or more of three crucial brain functions that correspond to the three major attributes of consciousness that are altered as its states change. The first function is activation, corresponding to the raised or lowered level of consciousness. The second is input-output gating, corresponding to the provenance of the information processed. The third is modulation, corresponding to the way in which the information is processed.

Because we can measure—or reliably estimate—all three of these brain functions, we can construct a three-dimensional model representing (1) the energy level of the brain and its component parts (Factor A, for Activation); (2) the input-output gating status of the brain, including its internal signaling systems (Factor I, for Information Source); and (3) the modulatory status of the brain, which is determined by those chemical systems that determine the mode of processing to which the information is subjected (Factor M, for Modulation).

When we enter the values of A, I, and M into the model, the state of the brain-mind—including its conscious aspect—is represented as a point in a three-dimensional state space. This point is constantly moving, and its location and trajectory are controlled by intrinsic and extrinsic influences. Using the AIM model measures we can—for the first time—begin to map normal and abnormal alternatives in conscious state onto a physiologically realistic schema.

This three-dimensional state space model has already had an initial application in studying natural sleep and its disorders. In this book, the principle focus will be upon those altered states of consciousness that are the consequence of two intentional manipulations of the brain system controlling conscious states. The first is the set of manipulations primarily affecting factor I, the input-output gating dimension of the model. This includes hypnosis, the relaxation response, meditation, and trance. The second is the set of manipulations primarily affecting factor M, the mode setting dimension of the model, which includes the psychedelic drugs, stimulants, narcotics, anesthetics, and mood altering drugs. I discuss the AIM model in more detail later in this chapter, and in chapter 7, where I fully explain its physiological basis.

Definition of States of Consciousness

Some scientists are sure that waking is the only state of consciousness worthy of consideration because only in waking do we achieve (1) veridical awareness of the outside world, (2) veridical awareness of our own conscious state, and (3) awareness that we have other awarenesses. Dreaming, then, is an altered state of consciousness, because all three of the unique features of waking consciousness are lost. We delusionally believe that we are awake when we are in fact asleep; we delusionally believe that we are perceiving a real outside world, whereas we are actually creating that world without benefit of external stimuli; and we are not capable of critically observing, assessing, and appreciating our delusional and confabulatory awarenesses.

Waking as the Norm

Although it seems obvious that there are states of consciousness other than waking, it does seem scientifically reasonable to take waking as the norm, the point of reference to which to compare other states of consciousness.

The irony is that we begin by choosing the most coarse grained parameters of waking consciousness because they are valid and because they are reliable. Alertness is one such basic parameter. It can be self-rated and it has easily measurable behavioral and physiological correlates. Alertness implies a high level of energy or activation, and it implies focused attention, usually on the external world. Internal stimuli, in fact, distract alertness if they arise unbidden when we are trying to focus on a book, an idea, or a conversation. In alert consciousness, the mind is in an expectant search mode and cognitive deliberations must be minimized. This is also true of meditation states and hypnosis when subjects self-activate large regions of their brains. Of course, there may well be many shades or flavors of alertness that our initial measures will not capture. Recognizing that our current measures are only temporarily adequate will help us remember to fine tune them as our maps of the conscious state territory become more detailed.

Two caveats arise, one methodological, the other functional.

Methodologically speaking, it should be clear that waking consciousness is itself a many splendored thing. That is to say, waking can be associated with an infinite set of conscious substates, no one of which is easily singled out as typical, stable, or even normal in a statistical sense. This is a problem to which we will return when we consider imaging studies, but it is important at the onset to stress that psychologists, physiologists, or philosophers have never subjected the vast panoply of waking substates to a detailed analysis.

Functionally speaking, we should not assume that because waking consciousness (whatever that is) is good at some things that dreaming (say) isn't, that dreaming is an inferior, degraded state of consciousness. Dreaming may be useful in ways not yet appreciated. Dreaming is certainly functionally superior to waking in fabricating a virtual reality. This imaginative, autocreative aspect of dream consciousness may be worth studying in its own right—not only as a way of understanding psychotic states as I have often suggested, but also as a way of understanding the highest functional achievements of consciousness in science and in art.

The two caveats come together when we ask if waking consciousness can be altered in such a way as to maximize the autocreative aspects so prominent in dreaming while returning enough wake state consciousness to critically analyze, validate, and report the creative product. The answer, still poorly articulated in mechanistic detail, is clearly "yes." By isolating the brain-mind, setting it on automatic pilot, and opening it up to spontaneous cognition and emotion, people can achieve a wide variety of goals, from literature (writing stories) to psychotherapy (writing stories about the self?).

Form vs. Content

Consciousness is always about something. Like a book, it has a plot, or like a film it has a scenario consisting, in part, of a script or a storyline. Like language, waking consciousness is often characterized by sentence-like statements, as well as by nonverbal perceptual monitoring, the contents of which usually go unremarked unless something unusual happens. In waking, the verbal channel of consciousness can be effectively dissociated from the perceptual channels. We say, "Don't distract me, I'm trying to concentrate"—meaning, I want to devote my limited attentional resources to cogitation (thinking is, after all, the essence of cognition) and actively exclude distractions that would interrupt the flow of thought by causing discontinuity. Whatever consciousness is about (content), it deals with that content in different ways (form). Whether internally generated content is consonant with the outside world or dissociated from it is one formal process. Whether associations between conscious elements are tight and concrete or loose and abstract is another. Whether the content can be thought about, actively manipulated, or remembered is another. All three of these formal aspects of consciousness are altered when waking gives way to dreaming.

Waking consciousness, whatever its content, can be controlled to help keep it on track. Left to its own devices, it might flit from external to internal stimuli and from one internal stimulus to another. Continuity (vs. discontinuity) is one example of this form of consciousness. A related formal property is congruity (vs. incongruity), which describes the coherence of the contents of consciousness at any instant. If continuity describes smoothness (vs. choppiness) of flow of the stream of consciousness, congruity describes its integrity, the compatibility of its components, channels, and elements.

As I write these words, I am aware of the conversation of my colleagues who have just sat down in the conference room and the click-click of my assistant's word processor outside my open office door. But by a mild effort of will I can ignore the content of their conversation and stay on the message of my writing. When the word "pregnant" enters my mind, I need a bit more of an effort to sustain my prose. Why? *Pregnant is harder to ignore than pizza.* Emotional salience is an aspect of content that interacts directly with the form of consciousness. Right this minute, I am not interested in pizza (because I just ate two hamburgers), but I am interested in pregnant (because my wife's period is two days late). Emotion is thus an important third channel of consciousness, even if it is often so subtle as to be ignored as the potent shaper of cognition that psychodynamic psychiatry and modern cognitive neuroscience have shown it to be. In waking, we are often unaware of any ongoing emotion in our consciousness, and yet a moment's reflection will convince us that we are always experiencing varying proportions of positive and negative emotion.

Because waking consciousness is so much the norm, we often forget that the content of the perceptual channel of consciousness need not always reflect the external world. This is still another example of the form vs. content distinction. If the percepts arise in response to entirely endogenous stimuli—as they do in dream hallucinations—the form, as well as the content, is likely to change. This is because it is more difficult to simulate the complexity of the external world than to copy it; when we hallucinate or dream, we need to create the stimuli that engender the images, as well as to perceive them. This may be one reason why it is so hard to think continuously—or even at all—when our consciousness is busy both cooking up and processing perceptual images. We have recently completed a study that shows this principle to apply across the five states of consciousness we assessed. That is to say, hallucinatory imagery and reflective thought are strictly reciprocal whether we are alert, awake, drowsy, asleep, or dreaming. The more imagery increases, the harder it is to think!

Why Distinguish Form and Content?

The first good reason to distinguish form and content is because the distinction is so robust. The second is that although the categories and exemplars of content are infinitely large, those of form are tractably limited. It is thus a simpler problem and science is wise to simplify. Beyond these methodological considerations, formal aspects of consciousness demand prior attention because they so often determine—or at least shape and limit—content (which is not to say the converse is not true, because content can shape form, too). Without meaning to be confusing, we must distinguish form and content because they are inseparable.

But the strongest reason of all for focusing upon form is because it is only in the domain of form that we have any hope of mapping from mind (form) to brain (form). Thus, in cognitive science we know the brain locus of word form analysis but have no idea as to how specific words (content) are analyzed. To ignore form is a bit like studying a language without considering its grammatical structure.

As far as altered states of consciousness are concerned, it is often the formal aspects that are emphasized: to have visions, internal stimuli must become predominant; to have intense visions, they must become very predominant, and when visions become intense, they are more likely to become exotic, numinous, or preternatural, and thus to suggest otherworldliness. And so on. To understand the visions of altered states, we had better understand how the form of visual processing is altered at the level of the brain. We have at least an odds on chance of doing this, whereas we have no chance at all of knowing why the visionary brain sees exotic flowers.

Formal Similarities of Successive Mental Images:
The Mushroom-Candle and Other Visual Transformations

The dynamic interaction of perception, emotion, and cognition in the creation of conscious experience is highlighted by the visual image transformations that are enhanced by natural and drug-induced alterations of brain-mind state. Later in the book we will read the detailed accounts of such transformations in the reports by careful self-observers such as Albert Hofmann (who discovered the psychotogenic potential of LSD) and Heinrich Klüver (who used mescaline to study visual hallucination). In Hofmann and Klüver's work, the most valuable descriptions are formal. That is, they emphasize form rather than content.

As a tribute to the autocreative capacity of the normal brain-mind and to our ability to appreciate and formally represent it I have asked my colleague Claude Rifat for permission to reproduce drawings that represent some of his visual image transformations. Rifat found that he could reliably induce elaborate visual imagery by voluntarily causing his brain-mind to enter the borderline states between sleep and waking that we will consider in more detail in chapter 5. By inducing such states, Rifat was opening the Dream Drugstore that is in his own head by purposely tipping his brain's intrinsic chemical balance.

Rifat made detailed sketches of his own to document many of the transformations that appeared in his visions. They all clearly reveal the principle of structural isomorphism (similarity of form) that others have reported. For example, a mushroom, viewed on end from the stem side down, becomes a candle mounted in an ashtray (figure 1.1). A child's snow sled, purposely rotated until it approaches head on to his view, becomes an axle with four men standing on it; this form gives rise to a fighter plane still coming straight at the viewer; the fuselage of the plane then turns into a rolled carpet and so on (figure 1.2).

The formal isomorphism of structure is sometimes also functional. Both the sled and airplane are vehicles and gliding frictionless vehicles at that. This same cognitive principle of formal association is clearly illustrated in the broad-bladed scissors that become a toucan's bill capable of opening and closing to cut and chop (figure 1.3). Life may unfold as images evolve. Just as in my ginger plant dream (see page 295), Rifat's

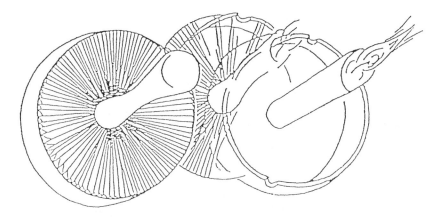

Figure 1.1

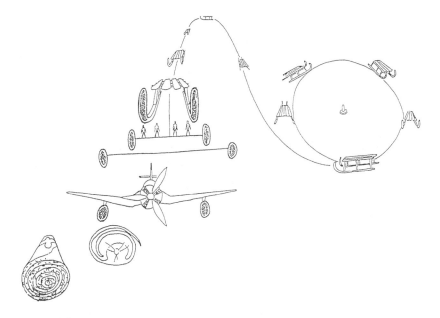

Figure 1.2

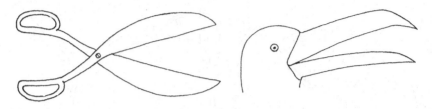

Figure 1.3

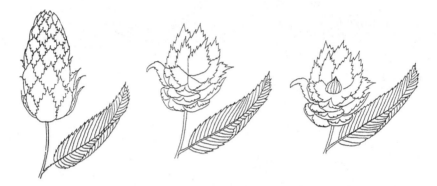

Figure 1.4

hop vine–beechnut "hybrid" tree bud gradually opens, and it then reveals a nut at its center (figure 1.4). A fuchsia-like blossom with Eiffel tower-like stamens opens and closes as its phallic metamorphoses oscillate back and forth between the botanical and the architectural domains (figure 1.5). More frankly sexual transformations interpose human and equine buttocks viewed in quasi-erotic locomotion (figure 1.6).

In other examples, a cornucopia becomes a pile of tires (figure 1.7), a crab bcomes a wineglass (figure 1.8), a keyhole becomes a champagne cork (figure 1.9), and a fish (again seen from the canonical head-on view-point) becomes a floral pattern stained glass window (figure 1.10).

To document these visual delights Claude Rifat, who was trained as a scientist in Geneva after his idyllic childhood in Saudi Arabia, made extensive sketches and notes, as part of his own effort to develop a theory of mind that could be related to basic science. But because he was not an artist, he asked Gilles Roth of the Museum of Natural History in Geneva, Switzerland to redraw them in the form shown here.

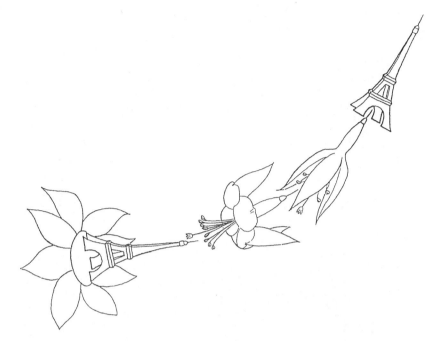

Figure 1.5

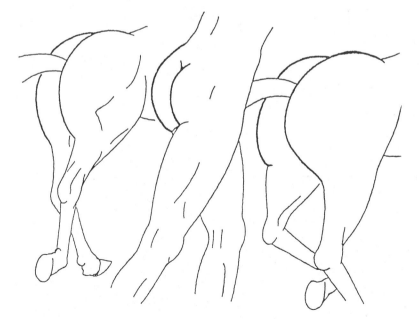

Figure 1.6

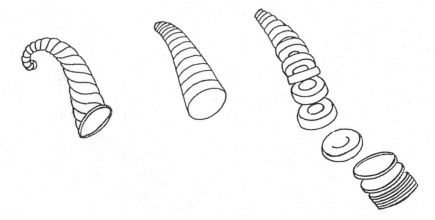

Figure 1.7

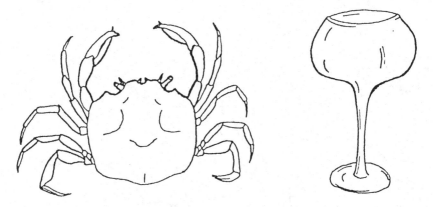

Figure 1.8

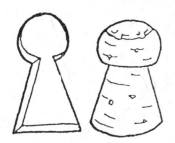

Figure 1.9

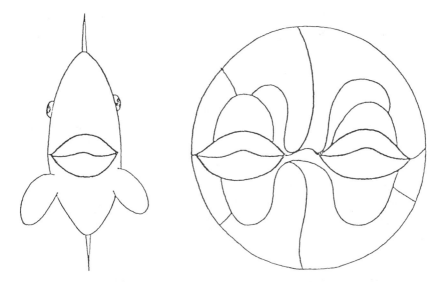

Figure 1.10

Like many of his contemporaries, Claude Rifat was drawn to experimentation with psychoactive drugs, but he soon learned that he could accomplish the effects he sought without them. Through his contact with the French psychobiologist Henri Laborit, he was inspired to elaborate models of these transformations that involve the natural neuromodulator serotonin, just as I will do in chapter 7. Claude Rifat's life has led him back to the east, but now it is the extreme orient that he calls home. There he has felt freer to pursue his self-observation based scientific inquiries and develop his personal, social, and ecological ideals.

Brain-Mind Concept

Is it possible to fuse the subjectivity of consciousness with the objectivity of brain activity? If the brain—or its informational content—becomes aware of the outside world and then of itself as the instrument of that awareness, it seems possible that the awareness itself is brain activity. We leave out the usual qualifier "nothing but" (brain activity) to avoid giving offense but that, of course, is what we mean.

Because we can't yet easily grasp exactly how this might be so but need to recognize the close interdependence of subjective experience and brain activity, I use the hybrid term brain-mind as a temporary compromise between dualism (which I reject) and monism (which I can't quite prove).

The word "interdependence" is important here because it allows that the subjective state of consciousness can alter the brain just as the state of the brain can alter the state of consciousness. In my brain-mind model, volition and automaticity are in dynamic equilibrium. Most brain functions (like other bodily processes) are automatic, but some (unlike other bodily processes) are reflective, deliberative, and decisive in altering the direction and content of subsequent mental activity.

The trade-off between science and spirituality is fair and square in this formulation. We need no longer invoke disembodied spirits to account for mental life. At the same time, we can retain the notion of free will that is the basis of our ethical codes, our laws, and our self-respect. Stretching the point, we can envisage a materialist spirituality. Because conscious states include poetic wonder, awe, reverence, and numinosity, and because we know all such attributes are aspects of brain activity, we can safely say that the brain is not only conscious, but is also a spiritual self standing in appropriate awe of its own complexity, creativity, and social conscience.

State-Space Concept

Brain-minds, like planets and many other heavenly bodies, constantly change their position in state space. In this view, our daily trajectory through waking, sleeping, and dreaming is orbital and obeys cerebral rules akin to gravitational laws. In fact, one of the most prominent rules, the circadian rhythm of rest and activity, is a clear adaptation to the geophysical cyclicity of light and dark, warmth and cold. This means that the state-space concept is not just a metaphor—important aspects of cosmic reality are built into the system at a very deep level.

The AIM state-space model describes the canonical alterations in consciousness quite well. But it also shows how little of the state space we actually use in our daily lives. Most of the zones of the state space are, in fact, forbidden. No trespassing signs are posted on domains such as hallucination, coma (irreversible sleep), and hypnotic trance (dissociations of the conscious-unconscious minds), and these limits are respected unless one tampers with one of the three dimensions of the space boundary. Brain damage may induce coma by irreversibly lowering the activation dimension (A). With respect to the voluntary alterations of conscious states, hypnosis may induce dissociation by altering the input-output (I) properties of the system. Psychedelic drugs may induce hallucination by altering the modulatory chemical balance dimension (M). As the system normally evolves over the course of a lifetime, a seasonal year, or a diurnal day, all three of the dimensions change, causing more or less time to be spent in more or less standard zones of the state space.

Historical Perspective

The phrase "altered state of consciousness" (ASC) took on its current narrow meaning in the psychedelic era of the 1960s. The meaning was centered on the spectacular and exotic visions induced by synthetic drugs like LSD, and was therefore strongly tilted in the direction of psychopharmacology. But consciousness has always been alterable and our present perspective has deep roots in the religious traditions of both Eastern and Western cultures.

Until 1953, physiology had very little of substance to contribute to the theory and practice of altered states of consciousness. Although Eugene Aserinsky and Nathaniel Kleitman's discovery that brain activation in (REM) sleep was associated with hallucinoid dreaming shook the dream theory tree quite strongly, it did not evoke the wider interest it deserved as the harbinger of integration between experimental psychedelism, psychology, psychiatry, and traditional neurobiology.

In retrospect, this narrowness is surprising in view of the foreshadowing of an integrationist doctrine in the monumental work of Sigmund Freud (figure 1.11) and William James (figure 1.12) at the turn of the twentieth century. Both Freud and James were by then already thoroughly persuaded that dreams, psychotic hallucinations, and quasi-religious visions all depended, somehow, on alterations in brain function. Their work foreshadows the central thesis of this book, that altered states of consciousness are the subjective concomitants of altered states of brain physiology.

How did the strong connection between these two great thinkers separate, and why did their messages get discontinued as the twentieth century moved, at its close, inexorably toward a vindication of both of them?

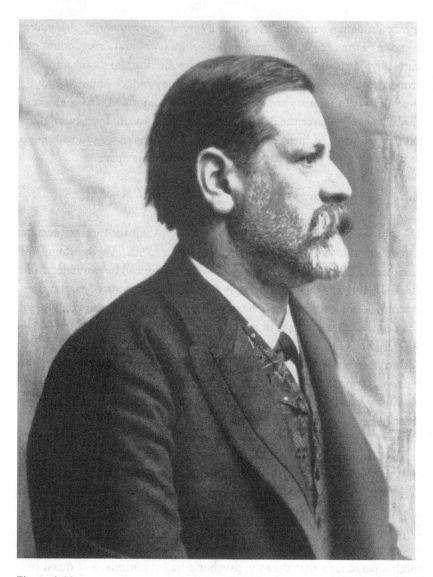

Figure 1.11
The Viennese neurologist and psychiatrist Sigmund Freud was an imaginative theorist who created psychoanalysis when his dream of a scientific psychology built on the foundation of brain science had to be abandoned. Dreaming was the altered state of consciousness that Freud tried first to explain in psychoanalytic terms. This is because the concepts that became foundational for psychoanalysis via Freud's masterpiece, *The Interpretation of Dreams* (1900), are the direct intellectual descendents of the key ideas in the failed Project for a Scientific Psychology (1895). By equating what he took to be the psychodynamics of dream formation

Freud and James were both children of their age, sharing a fascination with the burgeoning brain sciences. Freud went even further than James had done in his *Principles of Psychology* (1890) when, in his *Project for a Scientific Psychology* (1895), he focused attention not just upon the brain as the organ of the mind, but upon its constituent neurons, their organization as circuits, and the flow of information within them as the physical basis of normal and aberrant consciousness.

By the time that they met in Worcester, Massachusetts, in 1909, Freud and James were giants, understandably wary of each other's fame but also surprisingly at odds with respect to the role of neuroscience. Having devoted his postgraduate career to physiology, Freud tried his best to evolve a brain-based approach to psychology but soon realized that not enough was then known to succeed. Following his disappointment with the *Project*, Freud had written *The Interpretation of Dreams* (1900) and most of the other seminal works of psychoanalysis as contributions to a new psychology of the unconscious mind that might someday be explained neurologically but which was, meanwhile, determinedly independent of brain science. This line of fracture split Freud's later work from its origins in neurobiology.

Because he never expected quite so much of it, James did not become disenchanted with neurology. Even in his 1912 *Varieties of Religious Experience,* he still maintained that the phenomena of greatest interest must have their roots in altered brain function. What bothered James was Freud's abandonment of neurology as his invocation of dynamically repressed unconscious grew stronger, especially as articulated in Freud's theory of dream symbolism and interpretation, a doctrine that James regarded as both scientifically unfounded and methodologically dangerous.

The kinds of differences that separated James and Freud led to schisms within psychology (which abandoned both Jamesian and Freudian phenomenology in favor of behaviorism) and in psychiatry (which turned away from neurology in favor of psychoanalysis). For fifty years, more

with all neurotic and psychotic symptom formation, Freud built a house of cards that is now tumbling down. Modern sleep and dream sciences now have the opportunity and the responsibility of restructuring psychodynamic psychology from the bottom up. (Reprinted by permission of the Archives of the History of American Psychology, The University of Akron)

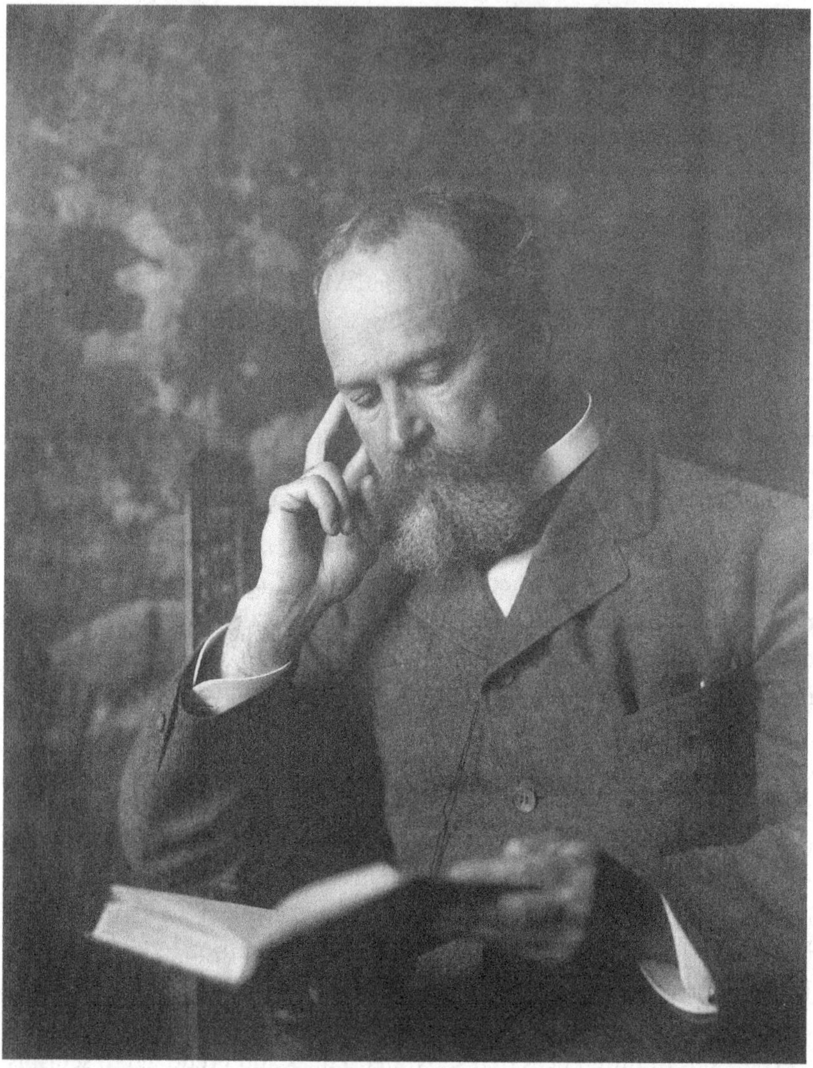

Figure 1.12
The American psychologist William James was an integrative visionary. Equally
comfortable in the domains of phenomenology and physiology, he is best known
as the architect of the philosophy of pragmatism, which attributes truth value to
the efficacy of ideas. Although James was scientifically rigorous in his attempts
to account for altered states of consciousness in terms of neurobiology, he
maintained an open-minded toleration of the spiritual, the mystical, and even the
occult. Early in his career James devoted fourteen years to the writing of his two-
volume masterpiece, *The Principles of Psychology*, published in 1890 when he

or less, psychiatry, neurology, and psychology went their separate ways. Today they are coming together again as cognitive neuroscience.

During the first half of the twentieth century, subjective experience—both natural and drug-induced—was declared off limits to psychology. The 1953 discovery of REM sleep opened the door to a reconsideration of dreaming and other naturally altered states of consciousness that occurred in mental illness. This discovery coincided with a rise in amateur experimentation with drugs that altered waking consciousness.

The psychedelic movement was a spin-off of psychopharmacology, which, in the 1950s, was producing the selective antipsychotic medication that would, by the end of the twentieth century, contribute to the closing of the state mental hospitals. Some of the drugs produced by the pharmaceutical industry were inadvertently psychotogenic.

That meant that both Freud and James had been correct in predicting that hallucinations and delusions could be chemically mediated, but it remained to specify how altered chemistry could lead to altered consciousness. The 1953 discovery of REM sleep and its associations with dreaming promised to provide an answer. If the hallucinations and delusions of normal dreaming were themselves chemically mediated, we could compare that chemistry with the chemistry of psychosis and the chemistry of psychedelic visions.

The brain mechanisms linking these three phenomena are the neuromodulatory systems of the brain stem, whose discovery began in the 1960s and whose neurobiological exploration is still a growth industry today. I still remember the excitement in Vernon Mountcastle's voice when he told me of "the brain within the brain" before Floyd Bloom's lecture at the first meeting of the Society for Neuroscience in Washington, D.C., in 1970. There were about 350 people in attendance, and many doubted the viability of the offshoot organization. Now there are 28,000 members, many of whom are ready for the next offshoot!

Not everyone believes that consciousness itself is within our grasp; however, few today doubt that we can alter consciousness dramatically

was forty-eight years old. Twenty-two years later, his Gifford Lectures appeared as *The Varieties of Religious Experience,* a veritable compendium of altered state disruptions, again analyzed in terms of altered brain function. (Reprinted by permission of the Houghton Library, Harvard University) and explain how the changes are engineered, even if we still don't know exactly what consciousness is and exactly how the brain manages to make it.

Psychopharmacology

Drugs had long been seen as a means of normalizing consciousness when its perceptual, affective, or emotional balance was tipped in the direction of psychosis and/or disabling anxiety. But prior to 1955, most of the drugs that were tried were nonspecific brain depressants like chloral hydrate, bromine, and the barbiturate sedatives. By reducing the brain's activation level, these drugs reset all of the molecules of consciousness simultaneously and unselectively.

At a Beacon Hill dinner party in the early 1960s, I was astonished to learn from a lady who suffered from severe and disabling manic psychosis that her trusted antidote was a so-called "sleep" cure. Her manic attacks were predictably periodic; they were also cyclonic. With her judgment severely impaired, my informant indulged in wild spending sprees, embarrassed herself in a rash of social indiscretions, and exhausted the patience of her very supportive family. So when she felt an attack coming on, she checked into her private clinic and was put to sleep for a month by frequent and regular injections of Seconal! She believed that the manic attack ran its course under the protective cover of drug sleep. But what a price to pay for protection! It's a bit like putting your legs in a cast to avoid getting blisters when you play tennis. You don't get the blisters, but you don't play tennis, either.

By then I had heard about Thorazine, the antipsychotic drug that ushered in the modern era of psychopharmacology. So I told my friend the story of its serendipitous discovery by Jean Delay, a French psychiatrist who was investigating antihistaminic cold medicines. Now, as anyone who has used them for motion sickness or allergies can attest, antihistamines are sedatives. As it turns out, however, phenothiazine drugs (such as Thorazine) also antagonize dopamine, a brain chemical system that modulates movement and thought so as to produce a related "tranquil" state of mind and body. Tranquilization is the reduction of anxiety without undue sedation. Its discovery rendered the "sleep cure" obsolete overnight.

Instead of knocking the patient out, the new generation of effective psychopharmacologic drugs all play upon the specific brain chemical systems that modulate the activity process and shape its conscious components. Some, like Prozac, affect mainly serotonin. Others, like Ritalin, mainly affect dopamine. Put another way, they play on the same systems that modulate normal consciousness so that in one activated state, waking, we do not hallucinate, whereas in another, dreaming, we do. The difference is in the modulation, not the activation! This difference permits a wake cure, creating a therapeutically desirable waking consciousness.

The late, great neuroanatomist Walle Nauta said that a thought was a movement not connected to a motorneuron. That pithy epigram captures the hunch of many of us that thoughts are virtual movements. In that view, psychotic thoughts are virtual movement disorders, which may be why patients so often pay with Parkinsonism for control of their psychosis.

The Psychedelic Revolution

In retrospect, tampering with the brain's own conscious state control systems was bound to influence the natural complement of therapeutic psychopharmacology that is recreational psychopathology! Prior to the pharmaceutical era, psychedelic chemicals were discovered accidentally, usually by making concoctions of plant leaves, stems, fruits, or seeds. Their chemistry and the mechanisms of the action on the brain were unknown.

Psychedelics alter consciousness in psychopathological directions, but because they are (mostly) reversible, they constitute round-trip tickets to and from forbidden zones in brain-mind space. There are good trips and bad trips. Good trips are characterized by altered perceptions and enhanced mood; bad trips by altered perceptions, fear, anxiety, and depressed—or violent—mood. LSD, the psychedelic drug par excellence, can cause both good and bad trips, depending on the individual taking it, the expectations and context of the taker, and the dose and purity of the LSD.

As is now well known, the potent psychogenic properties of LSD were discovered by the Swiss chemist Albert Hofmann, who was synthesizing molecules for Sandoz Laboratories. In 1938, Hofmann was making drugs with structural similarities to ergot, a naturally occurring chemical with strong effects on the vascular system. LSD-25 was one of Hofmann's creations. But it was not until 1943 that Hofmann had the variety of religious experience later sought by many users of the drug. That was the good trip. But he also had a psychosis. That was the bad trip.

As with Thorazine, this discovery was both serendipitous and perspicacious. And, as with Thorazine, LSD's mechanism of action turned out to be related to the neuromodulators. In this case it was serotonin that was blocked, but dopamine transmission was also affected. The prominent effect on dopamine was *activation*. Recent work on serotonin-dopamine interaction suggests that serotonin may inhibit dopamine function such that a decrease in serotonin efficacy leads indirectly to dopamine enhancement. This combination of serotonin blockade and dopaminergic enhancement is interesting because it mimics the chemistry of REM sleep in which normal dreaming occurs.

This suggested an analogy between LSD's mind-altering effects and normal dreaming, leading many of us to hypothesize a common physiological mechanism by which LSD might push the waking brain in the direction of REM. But, as I learned to my great disappointment in 1961, LSD does not enhance REM sleep when given to animals. On the contrary, it produces the same intense arousal and agitation that Hofmann describes so well. Only if it is injected during the natural transition from NREM sleep to REM is it able to potentiate the REM production system.

These findings together suggest that LSD psychosis is a dreamlike state that occurs in waking and that dreaming is an LSD-like state that occurs in sleep. It is in this sense that dreaming is properly regarded as an altered state of consciousness with mechanistic and subjective similarities to the narrowly defined ASCs of the psychedelic era.

Dreaming, Psychosis, and Psychedelicism: Analogy or Identity?

I am arguing so strongly for an analogy between these three altered states of consciousness as to risk being seen as espousing identity. Let me set the record straight in two important respects. First, the phenomenology, although formally similar, is distinctive in each case. Second, the mechanisms—which are still only very partially understood—are also distinctly different.

With respect to the phenomenology, it is clear that both psychedelicism and psychosis are altered states of waking, whereas dreaming is an altered state of sleep. That means that many aspects of cognition and especially working memory are preserved in those conditions associated with waking. This allows self-observation and even insight, which are highly desirable features in the integration of the voluntary drug experience and in the attempt to cope with psychosis. But is this difference qualitative? Sometimes, even usually, the answer is yes. But sometimes, however rarely, we can recover working memory while dreaming, become lucid, and watch the psychedelic/psychotic show!

As far as the mechanisms are concerned, we know that they are different in important respects. The psychedelic drugs are exogenous, whereas the brain chemicals mediating dreaming and psychoses are endogenous. And although the brain chemicals that are altered in dreaming and psychosis may be similar—or even the same—the ways in which they are altered must be quite different. Here again, we might suppose that some, or even most, of these mechanistic differences are qualitative. But if even some are only quantitative, then the borderline between analogy and identity really does break down.

Time will tell how far the analogy can be pushed. For now, it is enough if I can convince you that it is heuristically valid. That goal will be achieved whether you feel enlightened or simply stretched in your thinking about these fascinating phenomena.

It is the main goal of this book to explore, develop, and defend that thesis from the scientific, cultural, and aesthetic points of view. The larger implication of this goal is to promote the concept of a unified theory that could account for all spontaneous and induced alterations of consciousness, whether they are produced and experienced in the context of natural life, scientific experimentation, therapeutic treatment, or recreational use.

2

Pushing the Envelope: How States of Consciousness Alter

In New England, farmers say, "If you don't like the weather, wait a minute!" Meaning, of course, that New England weather is constantly changing. This is like the brain and its mind. The easiest way to alter your consciousness is to wait a minute, or an hour. And if this subtle but robust gradation of change in consciousness doesn't satisfy you, wait 12 hours and, if it is afternoon when you start counting, you will surely notice something profound occurring around midnight. By then, you are very likely to be unconscious!

This is all another way of saying that consciousness alters spontaneously. But because unconsciousness is not what psychedelic adventurers usually lust after, you may have to wait another six hours for a dramatic change. By then your consciousness will almost certainly be altered in a clearly psychedelic direction. Whether you know it or not, you are likely to dream for at least one hour per day, and the likelihood of awakening spontaneously from a dream goes up to about 50 percent by 6:00 A.M.

This morning, it was 6:30 A.M. when I awoke, just having looked into the largest and most spectacular underground limestone cavern that I have ever seen. A luminous light like that which is seen in the moments after a thunderstorm filled the space and lit up the zillions of stalactites that decorated the cavern's dome-like ceiling. The dizzying sense of a hungry gulf opening up beneath me was at once terrifying and fascinating, and I was dangerously close to the precipitous edge of the cavern opening even as I was simultaneously driven back from its engulfing lip. Flushed with this mix of anxiety and elation, I broke from the grasp of this approach-avoidance seizure by waking up.

This scenic development in my dream resolved a problem that had begun (to the best of my poor recollection) about two scenes back, when I was asked what I meant by "article shelf" in reference to a wide board that had been nailed to a log. I frankly couldn't remember ever having used that phrase but said, after a moment's hesitation, "It is a shelf that you can put articles on," and was quite satisfied by this explanation.

But none of the dialogue made any sense to the immediately ensuing dream action, in which there was the now shelfless log and another big log that I was struggling with in a vain effort to prevent them both from rolling down a steep incline. As they slipped from my grasp and careened down the hill, my anxiety mounted until they kerplopped into the small pond at the bottom of the hill. What a relief it then was to notice that I could retrieve at least one of them by wading into the shallow pond edge.

As I started to go down the slope, I was astonished to see the pond water begin to churn and to see the logs stand up on end in an impossible defiance of gravity and several other rules of physical mechanics! Of course, the most obvious explanation of this experience—that I was in an altered state of consciousness—never occurred to me. Instead, and this is the resolution I spoke of above, the earth opened up and the pond water and the logs slid through the aperture into the psychedelic cavern that opened my story. "It's a limestone cavern," I exclaimed to no one in particular as I ran down to examine its vast and exotic volume.

Spontaneous Alterations

As far as I know, this alteration in my consciousness happened spontaneously. And I have no idea, even in retrospect, what if anything in my recent experience stimulated or was—even symbolically—represented by it. All I know is that any time I begin to write about dreams, my awareness of them increases. Because this book is about the psychedelic potential of dreams, it is certainly possible that my brain-mind is primed to produce exotic imagery. But I did not prime it explicitly as I do sometimes when I want to have a specific kind of exotic dream or become lucid and enjoy watching a dream unfold with half of my brain-mind dissociated from REM and bumped up into waking consciousness.

Instrumental Alterations

In contrast to completely unanticipated dreams such as the example just given, my conscious self-priming of, say, kaleidoscopic dream imagery is instrumental and my own brain-mind is the instrument! In other words, I make the conscious decision to alter my future state of consciousness by a deliberate and specific autosuggestion. And it works. What other evidence do we need to convince us that consciousness is causal? What other evidence do we need to accept the robust reality of free will?

But because our dreams have minds of their own, our ability to control our own consciousness is limited and we may want to resort to an accomplice. Accomplices can be other people like therapists or hypnotists who hold us to a task or even push us in one direction or another, or they can be physical devices like our Nightcap, which records sleep and can be programmed to wake us up according to the time elapsed in one or another stage of sleep. I will describe how the Nightcap works in Chapter 3.

Or we could take a drug like LSD, or Prozac, and expect dramatic alterations in consciousness. These drugs are effective because they speak the brain's own chemical language. Although it is precisely this drug-brain dialogue that will be prominently featured in this book, that is not to say that I advocate drug-taking. In fact, I admit to a deep-seated bias against it. But we have learned so much from drug experiments that we need to know about them even if we prefer more natural, physiological, and psychological techniques. It is my fond hope that this book might even be an instrument of conscious state alteration.

Psychological Instruments

Autosuggestion is one of the most potent techniques for altering consciousness. Everyone knows the joke about telling the self to stop thinking about elephants. It doesn't work. But priming does work, and it works in two ways that are particularly relevant to the altered states agenda of this book. Cognitive scientists interested in memory have studied priming extensively. It is frequently defined as the biasing of networks within the brain during associative learning so that semantic meanings can be linked.

The linking facilitates retrieval of semantically related words. As such, it is essential to comprehending reading and speech.

But the brain can be primed in more general and more easily understood ways. It can be put on automatic search for words or ideas. One can use priming to increase the probability of remembering dreams, of being able to observe dreaming as it unfolds, and of being able to select or change the plot of dreams more or less at will. This is an interaction between the automatic state control system in the brain stem that, like a theatrical production, prepares the stage set of consciousness for dramatic action and the playwright-director in the more voluntary upper stories of the brain who chooses the plot, assigns the characters roles, and tells them how to act. Or, in an analogy with computer processes, priming the brain to achieve complex results is a bit like loading a program.

Of course, the brain is never so neatly programmed in dreaming. Even when one specifies a dream action, such as flying, details like one's trajectory, vehicle, and observed landscape may be filled in—as if by chance—or may change without notice, as if automaticity was constantly struggling to regain the upper—or is it the lower—hand!

Relatively speaking, it is a bit like the power of positive thinking running up against unbidden doubt during waking. Andrew Carnegie, the Maharishi, and the Dalai Lama are all gurus of positivity because they charismatically project top-down power over negative emotions like doubt and fear that well up from the depths of most of their followers.

In fact, normal dreaming is not all that ecstatic precisely because, there too, negative emotion is an unchained demon spoiler of our fantasized pleasure. Increasingly, the evidence from dream studies indicates that plot details are often designed to fit the directions of anxiety, fear, and anger rather than joy, elation, and erotic pleasure.

Last night, for example, I was thrilled to experience the potent onrush of dreaming that often accompanies the reshifting of my sleep when I travel. After a sleepless first half-night, I began to dream intensively in the second half. In each of the three scenes I remember the emotion turned—or remained—painfully negative.

In the first scene I was riding on a train. I was seated on the aisle next to a companion by the window. We both had our backs to the train's forward direction. I was enjoying the speed of the train, the lushness of the landscape flashing by, and the excitement of the game that I was playing with my fellow railway-car passenger.

The "game" was to maintain my emotional equanimity—and, if possible, my sense of humor—as various tests of will and patience were administered. In fact, my dream train protagonist seemed vaguely like one of my foremost adversaries in the long-simmering debate about the contributions of brain science to dream theory! His provocations, at first gentle and easy to deflect with an insincere smile, became increasingly hostile and then downright sadistic.

Two brutal sorties stand out as I struggle to recall the longer sequence of which they were a part. In the first, his argument against me was accompanied by a straight-arm push-off (which I countered with a thumping punch to the body). In the second, he illustrated his discourse by the use of surgical instruments like hemostats and wound clips to pinch and stretch the cut skin.

"What is psychedelic about that?" you ask, incredulous. "It sounds horrible!"

It was horrible. But even though I was not fully lucid, I was dimly aware that I was dreaming and I was enjoying dreaming, even if I wasn't enjoying that particular dream.

In retrospect, I can now see how clearly and directly this dream reflects the reality of my intellectual situation. I say that dreaming is a brain-based state of consciousness whose features reflect the selective activation (or an inactivation) of the specific brain neurons and brain regions in REM sleep. Others maintain that dream psychology is independent of brain physiology—or at least anything known about it—and try, by any means including stiff arms and more aggressive personal insults to drive me off what they take to be their territory—or, in the metaphorical language of my dream, to throw me off their dream train!

But I won't budge. At some level, even in my deep REM rebound dream sleep, I am aware that my dream is a double vindication because it shows clearly how physiology and psychology intersect to form the general setting of the dream and how they interact to determine its particular dramatic form. So, yes, the wound clips really hurt, but, no, I don't really think they are real.

In the second dream scene, my wife Lia and I are in a hotel whose location and identity are unspecified. In reality, we are spending the first night of our summer vacation in the Hotel Miramare on the island of Stromboli in the Eolian Sea. Outside, a weather clearing storm is brewing and several cats in heat are howling. So, again, reality and fantasy are in a duel for control of my consciousness. Fantasy wins, but it cannot completely dominate the local realities of time, place, person, and—in this case—tempestuous weather conditions.

To get away from our dream hotel and keep to our travel schedule I am magically provided with a rental car. How wonderful! What a relief to be mobile! But what a strange car. It is a 1940s Chevrolet, heavy and flatulent, which audibly sucks gas when I press the accelerator. To rent it, I must sign a very disadvantageous contract in which I assume responsibility for every conceivable financial eventuality. For example, I must not, on pain of penalty, remove the white sheets from the dashboard and seats of my galumping Goliath of a dream car.

With typical dream exigency—in the face of complete disorientation— I drive out of the hotel garage knowing full well that I have no specific rendezvous with Lia, who is still in the lobby with the rental car agents, who are actually insurance executives. And although I recognize this to be an insane scenario, I am not conscious of the now obvious fact that it is a dream.

What is worse, when I exit the hotel I notice that I am lost in a complex maze of country roads only barely cleared of a deep recent snowfall. At several points I have to get out of the car and push it uphill through the snow banks. So, I am getting somewhere, but where I don't know, and only with a Sisyphean effort! Anxiety and disorientation—two of the cardinal dream universals that I attribute to REM physiology—are in league with the psychological particularities of our voyage, our hotel, and the wild weather to produce this transportation dream transition.

And then—to begin scene three—another dream miracle happens! I arrive at a splendid mansion that has been elaborately decorated with life-size comic characters of people painted on every wooden door and wall panel. Now *this* is psychedelic! Why? Because the colors are so vivid, the characters so lifelike, and so psychologically revealing. I am gushing praise to my hostess, a sophisticated lady with a long dress, when she says mysteriously, "You are always so subtle and so accurate in your recognition of deeper realities."

"What the hell does that mean?" I wonder. Then the answer comes clearly. I am in a mental hospital cleverly disguised as an avant-garde art hotel! And my fellow guests are all lunatics—the dour fellow who greets me like a long lost friend in the lobby is a melancholic. And one of my real-life patients is there too, and has written me a profuse and typically obsessive letter of greeting. I chuckle knowingly and wink in recognition at my hostess as if to say, "Why yes, of course. This dream hotel is really a high-class madhouse." This scene clearly makes another point that I have been advancing in debate-like dialogue with still another real-life colleague—in this case a charmingly friendly but still quite earnest opponent of my views. That point is that dreaming, psychedelic drug taking, and organic delirium all share a common chemical mechanism: an alteration of neuromodulatory balance.

So this dream scene, like the others, is a self-fulfilling hypothesis: dreaming is an artful illusion, akin to psychosis, a delightful madhouse whose form is universal and whose content, while particular in some respects, is greatly constrained—and shaped—by the universal forms.

Pharmacology

Enter the drugs themselves. By drugs, I mean those exogenous chemicals that, like the cats in heat on that stormy night at the Hotel Miramare, interact with the endogenous brain chemicals that determine the formal properties of dreaming. But in this case the balance of the waking brain is tipped in the direction of dreaming so that it becomes possible to hallucinate visually (with eyes open instead of eyes closed) and live out fantastic scenarios with people whose identities have the same plasticity as dream characters (though they may be real-life psychedelic co-conspirators). How does this shift in balance occur? The answer is that the brain has a built-in tendency to shift the dominance from one neuromodulatory system to another.

The easiest way to conceptualize the pharmacological action of psychedelic drugs on the waking brain is by analogy to this natural change in neuromodulatory balance from waking to dreaming. Any drug that interferes with the synthesis, release, reception, or enzymatic breakdown of serotonin, norepinephrine, or acetylcholine is potentially psychedelic—

and potentially psychonoxious! Just as it is impossible to predict whether a dream will be associated with pleasant (elation) or unpleasant (fear, anxiety) feelings, so it is impossible to know whether a drug will trigger positive or negative emotions. The distinction between pleasant and unpleasant psychic effects is an important one and as drug-takers well know, not entirely determined by the type of drug. Thus, depending on dose, setting, and expectation, LSD—like REM sleep—can cause "good trips" and "bad trips."

In using the term "bad drug trips," I mean to dissolve the artificial boundary between legitimate, medically prescribed molecules and such illegal recreational drugs as cocaine and heroin. I fully understand and acknowledge the need for control of the most dangerous—because most addicting—of these molecules. But this valid, socially determined distinction must not be allowed to lull us into thinking either that legal drugs are safe or that illegal drugs do not act on the same brain structures and functions as the legal ones.

Remember my dream train ride, my dream car ride, and my dream art hotel, each of which comprised good and bad trip features. The extent to which these features were "bad trips" is also a function of dose, setting, and expectation. When I travel, I become REM sleep deprived and I am quite naturally both anxious and confused about my new location. Last night, as I experienced these wild dream scenes (and two others as yet unreported), my brain was both paying back a cholinergic REM debt, and stockpiling serotonin and norepinephrine so that I can stay awake this morning and write this chapter with some semblance of coherence and energy.

Acetylcholine, dopamine, norepinephrine, and serotonin are members of the class of brain chemicals called neuromodulators. Although they do not themselves convey signals about content, the neuromodulators alter the form—or mode—of processing of the content. Drugs that alter waking consciousness interact with one or more of these mode-setting chemicals. Because these modulatory systems provide so rich a neurobiological foundation for building a unified theory of natural and artificial alterations of consciousness, we introduce their anatomical and chemical structures in figures 2.1 through 2.5.

If I were to take LSD now, I would immediately interfere with my brain's serotonergic neuromodulation and slide back into a more dream-

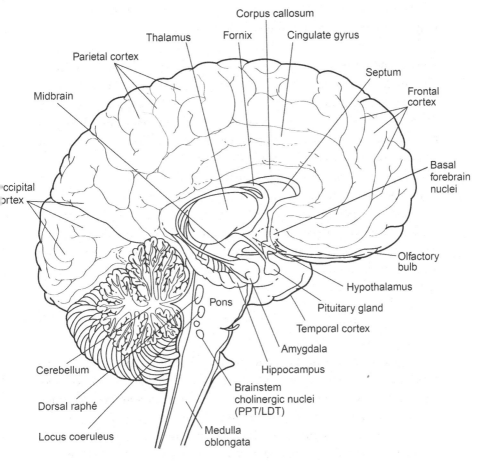

Figure 2.1
Human brain structure. This schematic sagittal drawing labels the main regions of the brain that are discussed in *The Dream Drugstore*. Subsequent figures (figures 2.2–2.5) illustrate the location of chemically specific brainstem neuromodulatory systems and should be compared with this one to identify the structures shown.

like conscious state. The tendrils of the wisteria vine outside my window might assume a surreal, serpentine image-aspect, and I might perceive their gentle wind-borne dance as a message from another world, at once sensual and portentous. Free of drug, I behold this scene as the welcome aftermath of the storm that rattled our windows for most of the night and that I can still hear in the relentless surge of the sea against the shore below my balcony. With my drug-free, REM saturated brain I can use the waving wisteria to tell my story just as the would-be poet could use its effect on his serotonin-blocked brain to tell his.

Pharmacology and psychology are thus in a three-way interaction with physiology that determines the form of conscious experience. That form shapes and constrains its content. And much of this process appears to be due to chance. If positive emotions predominate, my dream or LSD trip will be psychedelic and possibly even ecstatic. If negative emotions prevail, my dream will be more or less nightmarish and my LSD trip more or less monstrous.

Health and Disease

As soon as the consciousness-altering power of drugs like LSD was discovered, their relevance to models of mental illness was appreciated. Strangely enough, however, the three-way correlation among dreaming and drug-induced and spontaneous psychosis has not previously been emphasized. This oversight is particularly surprising because the formal analogy between dreaming and psychosis had been recognized for well over a century. Many pre-Freudian scholars such as Wilhelm Wundt specifically hypothesized a common physiology shared by dreaming and natural psychosis. The fact that drugs could produce dreamlike psychotic states in waking would seem to provide almost conclusive proof of the validity of this hypothesis and allow us to further specify it even at the molecular level!

Modern psychopharmacology has built its strongest base on the power of mind-altering drugs to influence the neuromodulatory system of the subcortical brain. One general rule that emerges from our studies of neuromodulators in health and disease is that of chemical balance. In many parts of the brain, acetylcholine tends to have a reciprocal relationship

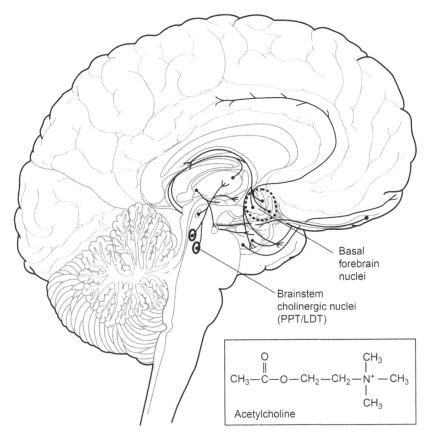

Figure 2.2
Acetylcholine neuromodulatory system. The neurons that synthesize acetylcholine (molecular formula in box) are located in the pontine brainstem and basal forebrain. The brainstem nuclei (called Ch.5 and 6 in Mesulam's nomenclature) project locally and forward into the thalamus, subthalamus, basal forebrain, and limbic system. The basal forebrain nuclei (Ch.1–4) project to the cerebral cortex and limbic system. Compare with figure 2.1 to identify structures shown. In this and the following three drawings, the very extensive and complex projections to the cerebral cortex are not shown.

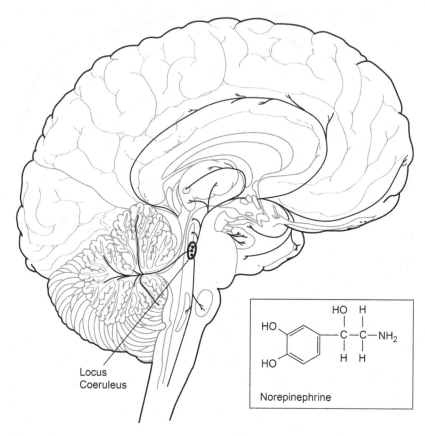

Locus
Coeruleus

Norepinephrine

Figure 2.3
Noradrenergic neuromodulatory system. The neurons that synthesize norepinephrine (molecular structure in box) are located in several brainstem nuclei including the nucleus locus coeruleus, from which axons extend caudally (to the
spinal cord), locally (to the brainstem and cerebellum), and rostrally (to the thalamus, subthalamus, limbic system, and to the cerebral cortex). Compare with figure 2.1 to identify structures shown.

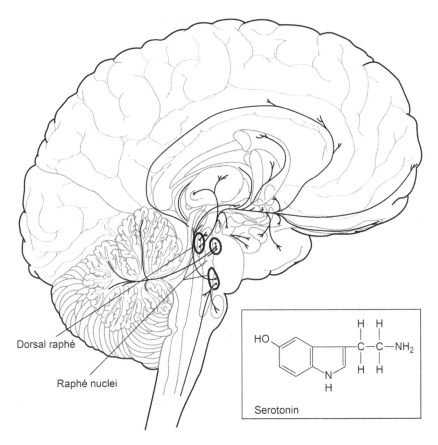

Figure 2.4
Serotonergic neuromodulatory system. The neurons that synthesize serotonin (molecular formula in box) are located in a chain of midline brainstem neuronal clusters (called the raphé nuclei). They project caudally (to the spinal cord), locally (to the brainstem and cerebellum), and rostrally to the thalamus, subthalamus, limbic system, and cerebral cortex. Compare with figure 2.1 to identify structures shown.

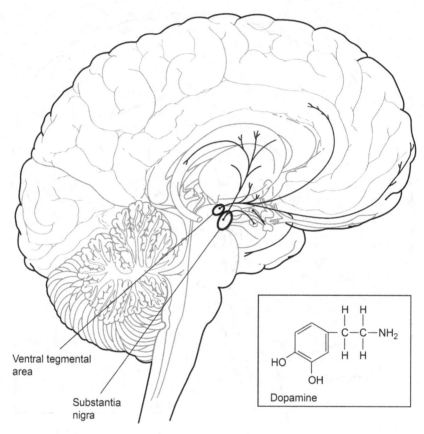

Ventral tegmental
area

Substantia
nigra

Dopamine

Figure 2.5
Dopaminergic neuromodulatory system. The neurons that synthesize dopamine
(structural formula in box) are found in the midbrain, from which they project to
the limbic system (the mesolimbic pathway), the cerebral cortex (the mesocortical
pathway), as well as to the extrapyramidal motor system (the nigrostriatal
pathway).

with dopamine, norepinephrine, and serotonin, but all of these systems interact synergistically to create the chemical background conditions of thought, feeling, and action. In depression, the beneficial effects of enhancing the synaptic efficacy of norepinephrine and especially serotonin (while simultaneously countering acetylcholine's efficacy) runs hand in hand with their suppressive effects on REM sleep and dreaming. This observation entails a powerful consilience of our models of mood control and dream control and is one of the most impressive scientific revelations of contemporary psychiatry.

In the case of schizophrenia it is dopamine, another neuromodulator not apparently involved in dream generation, whose overactivity results in psychosis and whose blockade by neuroleptics effects antipsychosis. We do not yet see how to fit dopamine and schizophrenic psychosis into the universal model, but hints as to how that might occur are already on the horizon. As the link between motor control and thought becomes better appreciated and the interaction of serotonin, norepinephrine, and dopamine is better understood, we will see, I predict, a seamless continuity among these control systems and their effects on consciousness.

One specific example will suffice—enhancing serotonergic synaptic efficacy can result in either a tolerable enhancement of dreaming (as is experienced under serotonin reuptake–inhibiting, or "SSRI" drugs like Prozac), or an intolerable enhancement of dreaming (as is experienced when serotonin-mimicking drugs like eltoprazine are withdrawn). In both cases the natural propensity to dream psychosis is augmented as a rebounding cholinergic system escapes from its drug-induced serotonergic inhibition that is in the service of improving mood.

Patients on either kind of serotonin-enhancing drug are being REM deprived just as I am when I fly to Europe. But instead of being allowed to recover—and experience intensified dreaming for one or two nights—they go on and on, night after night, dreaming endlessly (on SSRIs), or suffer such powerful REM rebounds (after eltoprazine withdrawal) as to continue dreaming after waking from REM. These hypnogogic hallucinations are no longer psychosis-like dream phenomena; they are dream phenomena that have assumed genuinely psychotic proportion.

The point, again, is that many, if not all, distinctions among dreaming, natural psychosis, and the drug-induced states are quantitative, not qualitative. However complex, the brain's own state control systems use a limited and self-similar set of molecules to program healthy waking and healthy dreaming. It is also already clear that alterations in the balance of these chemical systems, whether by genetic predisposition or such experimental misadventures as bad drug trips, can result in one of the three kinds of psychosis: organic delirium, schizophrenia, or major affective disorder. Thus the boundary between health and disease is as fluid and dynamic as that between dreaming and psychosis. Although I recognize that there are many important differences between these states and many details still to be established to understand how the boundaries between them are dissolved or maintained, the vision of a set of simple universal laws of consciousness is already in focus and we must seize the opportunity to sharpen that focus and extend the boundaries of that vision.

The State-Space Concept and a Model of It: AIM

The three-dimensional AIM model is a first attempt to develop a schema that could represent some well-known aspects of brain physiology and pharmacology in a manner consistent with the continuity and diversity of mental states. Activation, A, is the overall level of activity of the brain-mind. We can easily understand this first dimension of the model by an analogy to the volume control of any information processing device. It regulates the intensity of conscious experience, whatever its focus and form might be. Waking and dreaming are both highly activated brain-mind states. Most sleep is much less so. We can objectively estimate activation by quantifying brainwave (EEG) measures.

When the brain-mind is activated, it may be open to external information (waking) or concern itself exclusively with internal information (dreaming). Physiology explains this shift by the second dimension of the state space, called I, for information source. I varies from external to internal depending upon two processes: input-output gating and internal stimulus generation. In order for the brain-mind to process external data, the sensory input and motor output gates must be open (waking) and internal stimuli must be suppressed. In dreaming, just the opposite is the case: input-output gates are closed and internal stimulus generation is enhanced. We can measure the strength of I by quantifying postural muscle tone (EMG) and eye-movement activity (EOG).

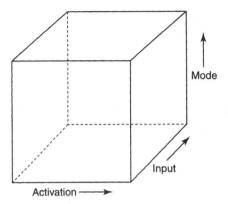

Figure 2.6
The AIM state space is defined by three parameters: activation (A); input-output gating (I); and chemical modulation (or mode, M). Activation (factor A) is an energy dimension that estimates information processing capacity and is measured as the inverse of average EEG amplitude and/or the rate of neuronal firing in the reticulo-thalamo-cortical system. It runs from low to high, from left to right, across the front of the state space. The input-output gating function (factor I) is an information source dimension that estimates both the capacity of the system to exchange information with the outside world and the capacity of the system to generate its own information. The I dimension runs from gates closed (front of space) to gates open (back of space). Conversely, internal information generation runs from high (front of space) to low (back of space). Modulation estimates the mix of chemical influences arising from aminergic (norepinephrine and serotonin) and cholinergic (acetylcholine) brainstem neurons (see figures 2.2–2.4). The M dimension runs from high aminergic (top of space) to low aminergic (bottom of space).

The third dimension of the state space model is M, which stands for modulation or mode. The M dimension, which we can quantify by measuring the strength of the brain chemical systems, determines the way that information is processed, whatever its source. The easiest way to understand M is to realize that it also stands for memory. The strength of M determines whether the brain-mind keeps a record of its conscious experience (waking) or does not (dreaming). M probably also determines the mode of associative processing, so that associations are either tight and logical (waking) or loose and emotionally organized (dreaming).

When we assemble the three dimensions, A, I, and M, as the bounds of a cubic space (figure 2.6), we can represent and visualize the continuous fluctuations of normal brain-mind state as a dancing dot whose each successive position is determined by the current value of the three measures (figure 2.7). Time is thus the fourth dimension of the model, which means that a succession of dots can represent the second-to-second, minute-to-minute, hour-to-hour, or even day-to-day changes in AIM. We can render these successions as lines of progress through the imaginary space that illustrate the regularities of continuous vicissitudes of conscious states (figure 2.8). For example, the cyclic recurrence of activation and inactivation during sleep reveals itself as an elliptical trajectory in the state space.

The three-dimensional AIM model is a first attempt to concretize and to visualize the state space concept. Because it has three dimensions, it *is* a space, not a plane, as are traditional representations of waking, sleeping, and dreaming. Furthermore, when realistic values are assigned to the three dimensions of the model—and with time as the fourth dimension—orbital trajectories of conscious state change emerge from the mapping.

The Margins of Consciousness

When we speak of "pushing the envelope," we refer to the normal boundaries of mental experience. Among the dimensions that bound consciousness are those of energy (determining high and low states of consciousness), of depth (determining access to unconscious processes), and of time (determining when one is high or low, shallow or deep). As drugs can alter all of these dimensions, we need to understand their physiological determination and the consequences of altering their determinants by psychological or pharmacological means. And these are only the concrete physical boundaries.

For many if not most humans the ultimate boundary, the ultimate envelope is that veil between the topical and the cosmic, between the sensory and the extrasensory, between the psychological and the psychic, between mortality and immortality.

For me, the first three are enough and sufficiently rich to keep me happily busy all of my earthly days—and to live on, if I am lucky, as an intellectual spark in the minds of my readers. But because so many of us long to travel out of our bodies, beyond time, beyond sensation, find other beings, reunite with the dead, or simply live forever, we will look at some of these yearnings, examine reports of their phenomenology, and

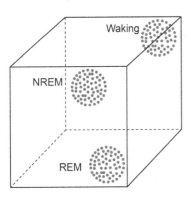

Figure 2.7
Normal domains of AIM state space. The domains of waking, NREM, and REM sleep are shown as cloudlike clusters of points, each of which represents the strength of A, I, and M at any instant in time. The waking domain is in the right upper back corner because activation is high, input-output gates are open, and aminergic modulation is high. The NREM sleep domain is in the center of the space because the values of all three parameters have fallen by about 50% of their range. The REM domain is again at the right (because as in waking, activation is high) but it is on the front wall (because the input-output gates are closed) and at the floor (because aminergic modulation has fallen to zero).

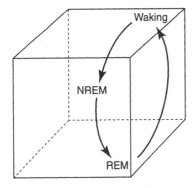

Figure 2.8
Normal sleeping cycle. As normal subjects progress through each sleep cycle the successive points of AIM follow the elliptical trajectory shown. The shape of the ellipse changes from cycle to cycle as subjects descend less and less deeply into NREM and more and more deeply into the REM domains. The rates of speed of transitions from domain to domain also vary: wake-NREM slow; NREM-REM rapid; REM-wake very rapid.

do our best, without being rude or insulting, to show how normal physiology can be structured to account for them.

One concept will prove particularly useful in this endeavor to unify our picture of the worldly and the other worldly margins of consciousness. It is dissociation, the process so aptly invoked and applied by Pierre Janet to hypnosis and to hypnoidlike somnambulism before being co-opted and sequestered by the psychoanalysts as a purely psychological phenomenon. In reclaiming dissociation for our unified theory of conscious states in chapter 5, I will emphasize its physiological instantiation. In this new vision, dissociation is the natural antonym of association, and like dreaming and psychosis, dissociation and association are in dynamic and continuous interaction.

In this view, dissociation is as functionally normal as it is statistically rare. One commonplace example will foreshadow this discussion. When you awaken in the morning, does all of you awaken fully and instantaneously or does it take time for all of you to wake up and do parts of you do it more quickly than others? Think of getting up in the morning and walking quite competently to the bathroom but once there feeling mentally sluggish, which makes you want to return to bed? And, if you happen to awaken—as I did today—in a foreign place, does it take you a moment or two to get your bearings, to know where you are and what day it is?

If your answer to any of these questions is yes, you already understand our natural tendency to dissociate—to be in one conscious state but to experience in it properties of another. I will show that when amplified this normal process can lead to such exceptional states as sleep walking and hypnopompic hallucinations, and that these exceptional states can become models for understanding out of body experiences, extrasensory perceptions, or alien abductions! All of these exotic experiences can— and usually do—occur in the privacy and safety of our bedrooms.

3

Waking and Dreaming: The Polestars
of Our Stately Cosmos

Last night I dreamed ebulliently at least three times, and in each of my dreams the theme was architectural, having to do with unexpected—but meaningful—alterations in the buildings of my life.

The first dream had to do with the dairy barn that I am restoring on my farm in Vermont. I was talking to Bob Limlaw, the master builder-carpenter who is doing the work. The second dream had to do with pipe leaks in my recently rebuilt farm house, also in Vermont, but all of the characters and themes referred to my laboratory in Boston, which badly needs remodeling now. The third dream concerned the bizarre and unique 1912-period office furniture that was being pilfered by my hospital colleagues as they anticipated the imminent closing of the Massachusetts Mental Health Center.

Between the time I went to sleep and the time I woke up my consciousness had somehow been reactivated, but it had also been radically altered. Because of these radical alterations, I was unable to connect my dream experience to my current whereabouts or even to recognize the bizarre content as a dream.

To have such vivid consciousness while asleep is paradoxical. Because the memory for dreams is so fleeting, it would be natural to assume that the dreams occurred in the instant before awakening as a by-product of the brain activation process causing me to wake up. But this hypothesis is incorrect, or at least incomplete. We know this because had I been sleeping in a sleep lab, instead of my bed at the Hotel Miramare in Stromboli, a distinctive constellation of physiological events would have preceded my awakening—perhaps by as long as 30, 40, or even 50 minutes.

My electroencephalogram (EEG) would have shown the sort of low-voltage fast pattern otherwise seen only in the most intense waking. That means that my brain was electrically activated, turned on, energized so that an extra-vivid form of consciousness was possible even though my behavior still superficially resembled deep sleep. I say superficially because careful observation would have shown that I was actually making small twitching movements of my fingers, my facial muscles, and, most dramatically, my eyes. In the sleep lab, electrical impulses associated with the eye twitches are amplified by the electrooculogram (EOG) and recorded as the rapid eye movements that give the brain activation periods of sleep their popular name, REM.

The REMs too are paradoxical, not just because they occur in sleep, but because they occur, together with the brain activation, despite a very strong physiological prohibition against body movement generally. This prohibition is recorded in sleep labs as the complete abolition of postural muscle tone, seen as a loss of electrical signals in the electromyogram (EMG). The range of EEG patterns seen in waking and the stages of sleep is shown in figure 3.1. Their correlation with muscle tone, eye movements, and the conscious states of waking, sleep, and dreaming are shown in figure 3.2.

When these three electrographic signs occur together in sleep, they are highly correlated with vivid dreaming of the sort I experienced last night. The stronger the signs, the more vivid the dreaming. In my case, the intensity of REM sleep may have been augmented by three factors: (1) the fact that I had experienced REM sleep deprivation in preparing for my vacation trip; (2) the fact that this sleep loss was aggravated by the trip itself, which forced my brain to change its REM sleep schedule, as well as adding to the REM sleep debt; and (3) the fact that in this idyllic setting I can sleep as long and deep as I like because I have few responsibilities.

The power of my dreaming was proportional to the power of my REM sleep—and that power was proportional to the power of my previously hypervigilant waking. It is this push-pull reciprocity—like the strength of the tide when the moon is full—that evokes the image of waking and dreaming as the poles of our conscious state cosmos. This reciprocity also mirrors a metabolic reciprocity deep in our brains that has functional implications we now only dimly perceive.

Each of my three dreams last night took an important element of my waking state of consciousness and altered it in surprising, amusing, and

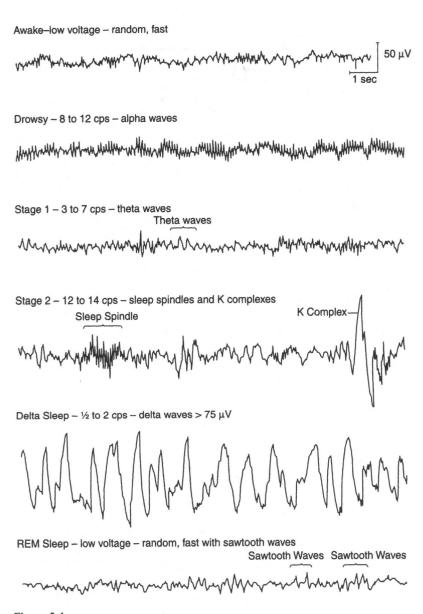

Figure 3.1
Human sleep stages. Electroencephalograms (EEGs) showing electrical activity
of the human brain during different stages of sleep. (From Hobson, 1998)

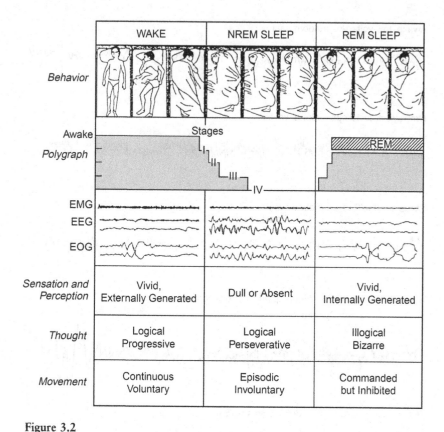

Figure 3.2

Behavioral states in humans. States of waking, NREM sleep, and REM sleep have behavioral, polygraphic, and psychological manifestations. In behavior channel, posture shifts (detectable by time-lapse photography or video) can occur during waking and in concert with phase changes of sleep cycle. Two different mechanisms account for sleep immobility; disfacilitation (during states I-IV of NREM sleep) and inhibition (during REM sleep). In dreams, we imagine that we move but we do not. Sequence of these stages is represented in the polygraph channel. Sample tracings of three variables used to distinguish state are also shown: electromyogram (EMG), which is highest in waking, intermediate in NREM sleep, and lowest in REM sleep; and electroencephalogram (EEG) and electrooculogram (EOG), which are both activated in waking and REM sleep and inactivated in NREM sleep. Each sample record is approximately 20 seconds. Three lower channels describe other subjective and objective state variables. (Modified from Hobson and Steriade, 1986) troubling ways. This bizarre but transparently meaningful alteration of content indicates the relative fixity of emotional salience and cognitive focus across the state change boundary that separates waking from dreaming. The persistence of mental and affective concern is not surprising. The places, the people, and the feelings involved all matter to me—they are the stage settings, the work projects, and the dramatis personae of my life.

What *is* surprising is the transformation of the visual images, the amplification of feelings, and the complete destruction of my critical self-awareness that distinguish my dream consciousness from waking. It is these formal features of conscious state change that we can expect spontaneous changes in brain physiology—or its chemical manipulation by drugs—to affect. It will be my hypothesis that the spontaneous and/or instrumental changes in brain physiology actually cause—in a direct physical sense—the formal changes in conscious state.

This hypothesis—which I consider already a scientific principle and wish to show you why—entails the concept of brain-mind isomorphism that needs to be explained. Let me outline the reasoning.

Visual Imagery

If I see a thing clearly in my dreams—be it my barn, the pipes in my house, or the post-Edwardian furniture of the hospital—my visual brain must be activated in such a way as to functionally approximate waking vision. Of course it can only be approximate, because my eyes are closed and my retinae are unstimulated by light. The fact that I see clearly in my REM sleep dreams—even though the images are ersatz variations of reality—means that higher levels of my visual brain—the visual association cortex, for example—must be active and must be processing internally generated signals in a highly integrated way.

The phrase "highly integrated" here means that time, space, and movement are all tied together in a convincing simulacrum of reality. In my dream, Bob Limlaw is showing me the barn work he has done while I was away. It is vast, extensive, and radical. I am alarmed to notice that not only is the wooden structure of the barn two to three times larger, but also that it has been subdivided into several building elements with interposed masonry segments (much like the architecture of the island of Stromboli where I am actually sleeping while having this dream).

"Highly integrated" thus also means hybridized, here indicating that my dreaming brain-mind is melding the architectural forms that I witnessed yesterday in my vacation setting with the unfinished work in Vermont. It is as if my brain were trying to arrive at a holistic unification of disjointed elements and suspending critical judgment in order to do so.

In one scene, I reconcile this discontinuity by visualizing a wooden wall of classic cattle barn windows that has been cleverly wrapped around a carved cement wall in order to hide it. In the dream, as I admiringly peel this wall away, it folds like an accordion door, even though it is 100 feet long! I look at Bob Limlaw approvingly and feel assured by the emotional integrity of our mutually respectful relationship. But I am getting ahead of my story by emphasizing the integrative power of emotional salience—which, of course, means that the emotional brain is activated, too.

Even though my retinae are unstimulated by light, we know from our sleep lab EEG recordings that my visual sensory brain *is* activated, and we know from our EOG recordings that my visual motor brain is activated, too. If we put two and two together, we can speculate that my dream vision is the sum, or perhaps the product, of these visual activation processes.

Because I don't much like sleeping in the sleep lab, I have worked hard on an invention called the Nightcap, which allows me to measure the visual motor of activation of REM sleep in my own bed. Had I been wearing the Nightcap in Stromboli during my Vermont barn dream, I would surely have noted an intense burst of signals in its eye movement channel when Bob Limlaw was showing me the architectural transformation of my barn's wall. The accordion effect would have been associated with the electrical signals registering the twitches of my eyelid that the Nightcap uses as a cheap proxy for the electrooculogram.

Back home in Boston, I have worn the Nightcap for ten consecutive nights as part of the first Nightcap study of dream recall following spontaneous awakenings of the sort that produced my three reports this morning. As I was getting used to wearing the device—which consists of a country handkerchief bandanna with a head movement sensor sewn into its forehead edge and a piezo-electric movement sensor embedded in a

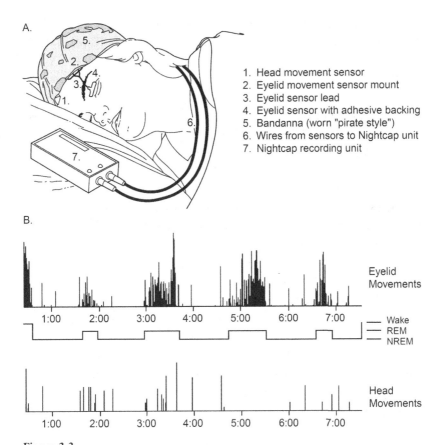

A.

1. Head movement sensor
2. Eyelid movement sensor mount
3. Eyelid sensor lead
4. Eyelid sensor with adhesive backing
5. Bandanna (worn "pirate style")
6. Wires from sensors to Nightcap unit
7. Nightcap recording unit

B.

Eyelid Movements

1:00   2:00   3:00   4:00   5:00   6:00   7:00

— Wake
— REM
— NREM

Head Movements

1:00   2:00   3:00   4:00   5:00   6:00   7:00

Figure 3.3
The Nightcap. Line drawing made from a photograph of a subject sleeping with the Nightcap. The eyelid movement sensor (4) is applied to the left eyelid and attached to a mount (2) located under the bandanna. The head movement sensor (1) is on the right side of the forehead, under the bandanna (5). Leads from the two sensors (6) travel around the back of the subject's head to the battery operated recording unit (7) lying on the bed covers next to the subject. Below sample Nightcap output and analysis. Top trace: Histogram plot of eyelid movements; second trace: hypnogram of computer-scored Nightcap data; third trace: histogram plotting head movements. The lower axis indicates the time of night. This example reflects the average quality of records, with an overall Nightcap-polysomnograph agreement of 295 out of 339 minutes (87%). (From Ajilore et al., *Psychophysiology* 32: 93, 1995)

Band-Aid-like tape attached to the upper eyelid (or see again figure 3.3)—my sleep was shallow and unrefreshing, there was little REM, and my dreaming was pallid.

After three or four nights, I began to have the expected REM rebound and I experienced truly epic dreams. These epic dreams are always associated with prolonged intense eye movement activity like that illustrated in REM periods 2 and 3 in figure 3.3. To my great surprise, some of these epic dreams occurred during the early part of an intense REM period that resumed and continued long and strong after I had dictated my report into the hand-held tape recorder that we had synchronized with the Nightcap recorder! Some REM periods had four or five mountain peak-like heaps of REMs in them, making me wonder how many spectacular dreams I had missed recalling simply because I did not wake up!

My Nightcap experience—interpreted in the context of more extensive and systematic studies—strengthens my confidence in the following isomorphic principles: dream strength and dream length are conscious state features that are proportional to REM sleep strength and length; REM sleep strength and length are isomorphically proportional to the previous wake state strength and length; and REM sleep dream content is isomorphically related to the previous wake state conscious mental content, especially emotionally salient content.

The fact that the visual imagery of my dream is synthetic and bizarre could itself be isomorphic to the autoactivation of the visual brain—to the near simultaneous activation of visual networks encoding general barn features, features of my particular barn, and the local architectural elements, cement and stone, that I was "playing with" on my walk last night.

Isomorphism dictates our finding evidence of visual system activation during visual dreaming. It also dictates finding visual system activation that is in some ways similar to that associated with waking vision but not identical to it. A corollary of this principle is that any drug that induces dreamlike visual imagery during waking will simulate the visual activation pattern of dreaming while still permitting wake state visual processing to proceed. The result will be a phenomenological and physiological hybridization of conscious state and brain state.

A detailed set of predictions regarding the physiological basis of differences between waking and dreaming is provided in table 3.1. Functional

Table 3.1
Physiological Basis of Differences between Waking and Dreaming

Function	Nature of Difference	Causal Hypothesis
Sensory input	Blocked	Presynaptic inhibition
Perception (external)	Diminished	Blockade of sensory input
Perception (internal)	Enhanced	Disinhibition of networks storing sensory representations
Attention	Lost	Decreased aminergic modulation causes a decrease in signal-to-noise ratio
Memory (recent)	Diminished	Because of aminergic demodulation, activated representations are not restored in memory
Memory (remote)	Enhanced	Disinhibition of networks storing mnemonic representations increases access to consciousness
Orientation	Unstable	Internally inconsistent orienting signals are generated by cholinergic system
Thought	Reasoning ad hoc Logical rigor weak Processing hyperassociative	Loss of attention, memory, and volition leads to failure of sequencing and rule inconstancy; analogy replaces analysis
Insight	Self-reflection lost	Failures of attention, logic, and memory weaken second- (and third-) order representations
Language (internal)	Confabulatory	Aminergic demodulation frees narrative synthesis from logical restraints
Emotion	Episodically strong	Cholinergic hyperstimulation of amygdala and related temporal lobe structures triggers emotional storms which are unmodulated by aminergic restraint
Instinct	Episodically strong	Cholinergic hyperstimulation of hypothalamus and limbic forebrain triggers fixed action motor programs, which are experienced fictively but not enacted
Volition	Weak	Top-down motor control and frontal executive power cannot compete with disinhibited subcortical network activation
Output	Blocked	Postsynaptic inhibition

From J. Allan Hobson, *Fundamental Neuroscience*, May 8, 1995 aspects of consciousness are listed in the first column, the difference in the second column, and the physiological basis of the difference in the third column. The balance of the book is devoted to a discussion of the basis of these predictions.

We are beginning to be able to check some of these predictions derived from the principle of brain-mind isomorphism. Not surprisingly, the visual system has attracted the attention of scientists developing new brain imaging techniques, including PET, SPECT, and fMRI. We know so much about the cellular and regional activation patterns associated with waking vision that it makes sense to focus on how the measurement of blood flow—the basis of brain imaging technology—maps down onto the neuronal level. This fundamental matching effort also provides the necessary reference standard for studies of vision during altered states of consciousness like dreaming and psychedelic drug-taking.

We have already had some surprises, and we are probably in for more! The early PET studies of REM sleep dreaming did, in fact, reveal selective activation of visual cortical areas as predicted by the principle of isomorphism. But the earliest stages of visual processing, which are located in areas V_1 and V_2 of the occipital cortex, were not implicated by the findings. Rather, it was higher-order unimodal visual association areas that apparently received more blood flow in REM than in waking. Our initial hypothesis was that dream vision might be built up, as it is in waking, from low-level neuronal signals of the sort that encode the external world in the retina and then are sent to the lateral geniculate body of the thalamus and on to the primary visual cortex (areas V_1 and V_2). This does not appear to be how dream vision is elaborated.

Vision through the retrospectoscope is always more acute than crystal ball gazing! Of course, we now say, why should we expect dream vision to be built up from retinal donuts and geniculate edges to fully sculpted 3-D images of the world? In REM, we don't need—and don't use—V_1 and V_2 for that purpose because, in fact, it is not at all from the retina and probably not only from the geniculate that the dream vision building blocks are coming. Interestingly, these PET findings are mirrored by those found during the visual hallucinations of patients with the Charles Bonnet syndrome, indicating that endogenous perceptions arise at high levels of visual processing. What do we make of this? After all, dream vision details are only *like* waking vision details, not identical to them. My barn is not really one built up on a visual edge-by-edge basis. In fact, the dream visual details have been radically altered—so much so that it is astonishing that I accept the dream barn as the waking barn—and in ways that only partially make sense from an emotional salience point of view. We still have a lot to learn about dream vision.

The most recent PET imaging studies are already questioning these early findings. Fasten your seat belts, there is an area of scientific turbulence ahead!

As for integration of vision with other sensory modalities, most of the studies agree about the implied hyperactivity of the parietal operculum, where vision, space, and movement meld so that we experience the world in 3-D as we fly through it (however turbulent the weather!). If we lose this multimodal cortical matching center, we lose dreaming altogether, whereas if we lose our visual cortex we still dream, even though we don't see any more in those dreams.

Emotional Salience

As happy as I was to behold Bob Limlaw's magical transformation of my barn (so happy, in fact, that I did not feel anxious about the architectural chimera that he had created), so was I *unhappy* to be unable to locate and control the pipe leaks that were flooding my farm house. This dream was a more typical display of confusion and negative affects, in particular anxiety and anger. In this case, the cognitive confusion and emotional discomfort made each other worse, not better, and signaled the unresolved architectural conflicts that I am currently experiencing with my laboratory colleague Bob Stickgold.

Bob wants to tear out the benches, sinks, and hood in our central work room and replace them with office furniture to better accommodate our burgeoning staff of junior associates, their desks, their file cabinets, and desktop computers. Knowing how much more expensive, hence valuable, wet lab space is than dry, I am resisting this change vigorously even as the pressure mounts. Bob says, "Just cut off the pipes and cap them," when I ask how he intends to effect the change.

Last night's second dream took place in Vermont, not Boston, but Bob Stickgold and his assistants were all there (as they often are when we have our lab retreats in the spring and fall). I am trying to stop the profuse leaking that is soaking the ceiling and walls when we turn on the water system. In reality, this can occur if the faucet drain caps are not replaced before turning on the water. But in the dream, the pipes are both cut off *and capped,* meaning that they should not leak. But they do leak. A lot.

I am running up and down stairs trying to solve the problem while Bob and his crew stand by impatiently and critically. At one point we are looking at a vast array of pipes that I find hopelessly confusing but somehow charming because they connote the amateur self-sufficient status of Vermont that I admire. I feel defensive and ask if the others do not appreciate the antique qualities of the house despite the bizarre and obviously dysfunctional plumbing.

"No," they shout in unison, "we do not!"

I soak this up for a moment and then retort, "Then why don't you get out?"

This scenario makes perfect sense to my waking consciousness. I have even imagined it, in a variety of forms, as our lab conflict has heated up. But so far I haven't spoken this out clearly while awake.

Isomorphism demands that my emotional brain has activated in parallel with my visual brain in REM. There must be some important differences between the pattern of emotional brain activation in dream one, when I was only slightly anxious and more elated than distressed by the strange visual alterations of my barn, and that of dream two, when I was very anxious about my inability to locate and control the water pipe leaks and furious about my co-workers' lack of empathy.

Until the advent of imaging technology we had no way of knowing what was going on in the depths of the human brain during normal states of consciousness like waking and dreaming. EEG probes of the temporal lobes of patients with epilepsy, although sometimes helpful in localizing seizure foci, did not indicate selective activation of the emotional brain compared with other regions during REM. But the imaging studies did show such changes, and they were the most dramatic, consistent, and theory-rocking changes of all.

Sigmund Freud must have turned over in his grave the day that Pierre Maquet and his colleagues in Liege, Belgium, told the world that emotion-mediating limbic regions of the brain lit up in REM! Here was the physiology of primary process thinking (read emotion-driven cognition) being scientifically demonstrated for the first time. We anti-Freudians were pleased too because—again for the first time—the human brain stem was shown to be selectively activated in REM just as it is in other mammals like the cat and the rat—and it was the same part of the brain stem too, a part called the pons. This meant that the cellular and molecular level findings on REM sleep control in animals might actually apply to humans, just as we had assumed.

Maquet's finding that the amygdala, thought to be the seat of fear, was selectively, bilaterally, and vigorously activated in REM has been consistently confirmed. In addition to the amygdala, the anterior cingulate cortex were also activated. Many think these regions are integration centers for emotion with other modalities of conscious experience like perception, thought, and movement.

An obvious implication is that emotion is in the saddle, as Freud assumed, during dreaming, but there is no need now to postulate disguise of the primitive emotions so churned up in REM. We need only integrate them with the conflictual issues of our daily lives to understand their transparent meanings, as in my broken water pipe dream.

What we *can't* yet do is say why in dream one I experience elation and satisfaction, whereas in dream two I experience anger and rage. Whether PET or fMRI will be up to this task remains to be seen. So far *all* of the REM sleep dreams of the brain-imaged subjects that have been studied have been lumped together. The next step is to compare the brain images associated with positive vs. negative dream affects. There are some early FDG PET findings by Gillin's group in San Diego that show a correlation of dream anxiety scale scores with lateral parietal and medial frontal activation.

Moving Brain Furniture

The PET and fMRI studies do, however, help us enormously when it comes to understanding the aspects of dream consciousness that are the result of losses of waking capability. Here I refer to those deficits in cognition, like poor memory, disorientation, weakened volition, poor judgment, and lack of insight that go with the memory loss. The vivid visual hallucinations and the exaggerated emotions are aspects and, sure enough, we find that brain hyperactivity is evidenced in just those regions that one would expect: the visual associative cortex (for the dream hallucinations) and the amygdala (for the fear, elation, and anger).

In all three of my dreams these features were prominent, yet I did not *notice* that my Vermont barn was so different that it could not possibly be my barn—even with the impossible alterations that had been made. Pipes in my Vermont farm house were a pastiche of the plumbing that is really there and the plumbing in my Boston laboratory. These glaring incongruities and discontinuities are the very essence of dream bizarreness. In waking, perceptions like this would cause such alarm that I would consider consulting some other psychiatrist.

My inability to take stock of what was going on, to direct my dream action, and to realize that my experience was entirely illusory denote the loss of critical judgment, self-reflection, and insight that we value so much as executive functions in our waking consciousness and without which we are as lost and helpless awake as we are in our dreams.

How could I not, for example, have recognized that the rooms I saw in dream three were entirely imaginary? No such rooms exist in the real Massachusetts Mental Health Center, where I have worked for the past 38 years! And how could I not immediately be suspicious that the furniture that I took to be vintage 1912 armoires and cabinets were the ersatz creation of my dreaming brain?

In the dream, I wasn't even shocked that respectable colleagues (like one who looked like Carl Schwartz but wasn't really Carl Schwartz at all) were blithely carting off credenzas to their own private offices. I might be a scavenger, but I am not a thief or a looter, even in my dreams! Or am I? Is my conscience dissolved along with my ability to be self-critical and self-directing?

No doubt this third architecturally bizarre dream is as typical and meaningful as the other two. Mass Mental *is* endangered. It *is* neglected. And, in the panic of political uncertainty about the future it *is* vulnerable to used furniture collectors—like me and the Carl Schwartz wannabes of our dreams! But this transparent meaning doesn't explain why the furniture was not veridical, why Carl Schwartz was still there, why he didn't really look like himself and—most of all—why I didn't notice all of these discrepancies and wake up to the obvious fact that I was dreaming.

Until the recent PET studies, the only physiological clue that we had was the animal evidence of diminished serotonergic and noradrenergic modulation in sleep. These chemicals, thought essential to recent memory processes, are down 50 percent in NREM sleep and nearly 100 percent in REM. That means that the brain, although electrically activated, is in severe aminergic deficit, so severe as to impair recent memory. Without recent memory, the perceptual and narrative coherence necessary to guide waking consciousness is lost. Here the principle of isomorphism is applied as follows:

No serotonin, no norepinephrine?

No recent memory (beyond the inertia of activation that enables me to recall as little as I do).

Skipping ahead to the psychedelic drug story, it would also follow from this principle that any exogenous chemical that interfered with either norepinephrine or serotonin (or glutamate and dopamine for that matter) might be expected to introduce dreamlike discontinuity and incongruity into waking consciousness. But we still need to account for the failure to notice them, to realize in the dream that things are wrong. What else is removed from cerebral capacity besides the ability to integrate, verify, and to remember our conscious experience?

We should have guessed that it might be the defective functioning of the dorsolateral prefrontal cortex, that part of the brain that is crucial for what the cognitive psychologists call "working memory." The dorsolateral prefrontal cortex is also thought to be the substrate of volition and of planning while the medial and orbitofrontal regions appear to mediate social judgment and insight.

The reason that we didn't guess that this region would be selectively underperfused in REM sleep is that the EEG shows no evidence of the implied deterioration. Why don't we suddenly see slowing in the frontal EEG in REM? Maybe such slowing *is* really there because it has been seen at sleep onset by Alex Borbely's group in Zurich. We should go back and look for it. To do so we would need to filter out the eye movement potentials that can be picked up by the frontal EEG leads, and we would need to use more sensitive tasks of relative inactivation, such as those used by psychologists like Richard Davidson in his studies of frontal cortex EEG activation asymmetry. It could well be that not only is the frontal brain less activated in REM than in waking, but that the left frontal brain is relatively more deactivated than the right.

How do the positive and negative aspects of the conscious state changes that distinguish dreaming and waking fit together? We can only speculate, basing our speculations on what we know about regional interactions under other experimental conditions. The first of these is the reciprocal interaction that we all know well to describe emotion and rationality. When we are hyperemotional (read hyperlimbic), we are hyporational (read hypofrontal). At best we rationalize. And, at best, we do that poorly. Does that sound like dreaming to you? It does to me.

In REM sleep we see this reciprocity at the brain function level. The emotional brain (amygdala) is hyperactive. The executive brain (frontal cortex) is hypoactive. Result: emotion is in the saddle. Rational thought is struggling—and failing—to get control of the runaway horse that is the dream. "Don't lose your temper," you say to yourself. This mantra says it all. If you can't maintain top-down control, your emotional brain will get the better of you.

It certainly doesn't help that in dreaming you can't organize your thinking because memory is so impaired. At least in waking you have the chance to gain insight via the embarrassment that accompanies self-observation in those repeated displays of pique, grouch, complaint, or whatever other negative affect drives your spouse and your friends away.

In dreaming you are not only out of control, you don't even know it! You can't keep track of the dream action from one dream to the next or even one scene to the next. I suppose that the three hokey architectures and the three kooky scenarios that I cooked up last night all occurred within one, or at most two hours. For all I know, they could have been my conscious experience of three episodes of selective brain activation/inactivation of a single REM period.

Yet what insight did I carry forward from one to the next? None! And this is particularly striking because I did wake up enough to recall considerable dream detail after each dream. But that instruction didn't help my poor brain learn. I was completely duped again and again the minute my pons, my amygdala, my perihippocampal cortex, my anterior cingulate, my visual association and parietal opercular cortices were revved up and my dorsolateral prefrontal cortex was muffled!

When I woke up, I immediately recognized that my previous consciousness had been dreaming *and* I was able to file away enough memory to
write these reports the next day. What *must* have happened? I must have
reversed the activation/inactivation ratio of my brain; and the PET studies say, "Yes, of course. That's exactly what happened!"

But now a nagging question arises. How are these sudden reversals of
regional brain function actually engineered? How is cerebral blood flow
diverted from top to bottom (in slowly moving from wake to REM in
sleep), and how is it redirected from bottom to top almost instantaneously
when I wake up?

This is an awe-inspiring question to which our answer must, for now,
be even more daringly speculative. To answer it we invoke an analogy
between the autonomic functions of aminergic and cholinergic neurons
in the periphery and their central autonomic functions (where they might
be expected to have a say in blood flow).

In general, the aminergic systems support fight and flight responses,
promote vasoconstriction, and direct flow to the muscles; cholinergic systems promote rest and recovery, and vasodilation. If this is true of the
brain—and especially the microcirculation of the brain—then it could
just be that the redirection of regional blood flow (that is measured in PET
studies) is caused, at least in part, by the selectivity ratios of aminergic and
cholinergic neuromodulatory neurons in the subcortical brain.

What I am suggesting here is that the mode of processing of forebrain
neurons and their regional activation patterns may both be controlled by
the neuromodulatory systems of the brain stem. These effects may be
paralleled in part by direct and indirect changes in regional blood flow
also caused by changes in neuromodulatory balance. If this hypothesis is
even partly correct, we would have two explanations for the price of one
fact. The concatenation of poor memory and poor cognitive control in
dreaming would be a conjoint function of a change in neuromodulatory
balance that alters consciousness by interfering with memory processes
globally (a metabolic effect) and with regional activation locally (a micro-
vascular effect). Fortunately, this hypothesis is testable and at least one
study has already affirmed it in the case of the cholinergic system.

Part II
Beyond Psychoanalysis: Toward a
Neurodynamic Theory of Mental States

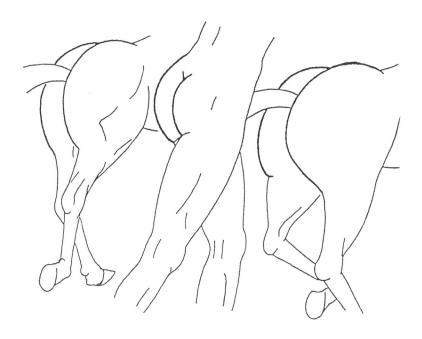

4

The Neurodynamics of Dreaming

In 1900, when Sigmund Freud founded psychoanalysis upon his dream theory, he was still heavily under the influence of the erroneous neurobiology of his *Project for a Scientific Psychology*, the work he abandoned in 1895. Because of this, the underlying mechanistic model of psychoanalysis and the practice that it justified was fatally flawed at the outset. The details of this argument have been amply described in *The Dreaming Brain* and are widely accepted.

The problem for Freud was that he did not know enough about how the nervous system was structured and how it functioned—especially in sleep and dreams—to root his theory in neurobiology. Now we do. In this chapter, I will show how sleep and dream science can explain the alterations in mental state that distinguish dreaming from waking in neurodynamic terms. In many cases these principles call into question the psychodynamic processes that Freud deduced to explain the same phenomena. The new neurodynamic view of dreaming thus forces a major paradigm shift in our view of how normal mental states are organized. In addition, it provides a foundation for understanding how drugs alter consciousness.

The main point of this chapter is that we can now recast psychotherapeutic attempts to alter consciousness in terms that are wholly consistent with modern neurobiology because the concepts that are emphasized are derived from that very source.

Alternative Models of the Mind

To help the reader grasp the impact of some of the technical discussion that follows, I here summarize the main differences in the two models of the mind that emerge from psychoanalysis and modern sleep science.

The essence of psychoanalytic dream theory is the *disguise-censorship hypothesis*, according to which already thwarted instinctual drives (id), trapped for safekeeping in the unconscious, are released from repressive control by the sleeping conscious mind (ego), and threaten to invade consciousness. To bowdlerize the id impulses and protect consciousness from invasion by them, the ego's censor neutralizes them by invoking the now famous mechanisms of defense, including condensation, displacement, and symbolization. This produces a radically altered a conscious state (the manifest content of the dream) that cannot be directly traced to its true unconscious origins (the latent content of the dream) unless a highly skilled psychoanalyst helps the dreamer, through a process called free association, decode (interpret) the dream. Thus the bizarreness of dreams is the product of a psychodynamically inspired charade whose function is to preserve sleep and keep the dreamer in the dark about the true motives of his maladaptive waking behavior, as well as his dreams! The dream theory is at the very heart of psychoanalysis, and its fundamental form is repeated in Freud's models of psychopathology and psychotherapy. If the dream theory is fundamentally incorrect, the whole psychological structure that is based upon it comes tumbling down.

Activation-synthesis is the hypothetical model that Robert McCarley and I first proposed in 1977 as a replacement theory for disguise-censorship. Activation-synthesis shares with psychoanalysis the conviction that understanding dreaming is a key building block of any psychological theory of mental illness. Activation-synthesis shares the conviction that dreams are of great value to the individual seeking to understand the interaction between (mostly) unconscious emotional impulses and (sometimes) conscious cognition. But because it differs in almost every other important detail, the way that it dictates psychotherapeutic theory and practice is radically altered, as I will try to make more explicitly clear in chapter 16.

Activation-synthesis ascribes dreaming to brain activation in sleep. The principle engine of this activation is the reticular formation of the brain stem, just as it is in waking, but the chemical mode of activation is distinctly different. It is for that reason and that reason alone that dreaming and waking consciousness are so different. In waking, the noradrenergic and serotonergic systems modulate the activated brain. In REM sleep dreaming, they do not. It is in this sense that dreaming is an altered state of consciousness, akin to those induced by psychedelic drugs in waking, and it is in this sense that the brain is a Dream Drugstore. The brain stores its own drugs and it releases them—or puts an embargo on their release—depending upon the brain's natural, spontaneous, and health promoting states. The brain activation of sleep is, in part, residual—and hence wake-like—especially at sleep onset, and it becomes wake-like again in late night stage II sleep. But it is also dramatically altered by the switch in neuromodulation that so strongly contrasts waking and REM. Although the brain stem is a primitive structure, it is in no sense an id. The differentiated activation it generates cannot be construed as, or even likened to, unconscious wishes.

Why are dreams bizarre? Because, absent norepinephrine and seroto-nin, the cerebral cortex and hippocampus cannot function in their usual oriented and linear logical way, but instead create odd and remote asso-ciations—not because of censorship or disguise. Dreams are therefore inherently and primarily bizarre, and dream bizarreness is neurody-namically, not psychodynamically, determined. For activation-synthesis, both emotional salience and the cognitive mishmash of dreams are the undisguised read-out of the brain's unique chemistry and physiology. This doesn't mean that dreams make no psychological sense. On the contrary, dreams are dripping with emotional salience, even when they are cogni-tively delirious.

This "transparency" tenet of the activation-synthesis theory frees the modern psychotherapist from any compelling need to interpret dreams at all. Dreams can and should be discussed and examined for their infor-mative messages about the emotional concerns of the dreamer. At the same time, the transparency principle enjoins us from suggesting that *any* of the dream content is in the service of psychological defense! But activa-tion-synthesis goes much farther than this in informing psychotherapeutic theory and practice. This is because it acknowledges the importance to dream construction of the emotional activation in sleep that is also best understood as a function of REM neurophysiology.

When we speak of REM sleep activation of the limbic, paralimbic, and subthalamic brain—and ascribe such dream emotions as elation, anxiety, and anger to it—we may sound a bit Freudian. When all is said and done, isn't *this* Freud's id, getting stirred up in sleep and raising havoc with consciousness? Not at all. According to activation-synthesis, the activation of emotional centers is a physiologically determined event that cannot be identified with the Freudian concept of unconscious wishes, even if it does generate strong emotions with a strong impact on cognition and behavior. More importantly and more decisively, dream emotions do not cause dream bizarreness, because they are neither disguised nor neutralized by the dream thoughts. On the contrary, they collaborate with the dream thoughts in the synthesis of transparently meaningful dream plots of great interest to our psychotherapeutic explorations.

In the view of activation-synthesis, the dream is its own interpretation. This is because the manifest and the latent content—like Freud's antique neurobiology and psychoanalytic dream theory—are one and the same! Not only is it erroneous and unjustified to interpret dreams according to the Freudian disguise-censorship rubric, but such a perverse practice also risks erroneous interpretation, as well as it risks ignoring the robust truth of the dream's transparent emotional salience. The modern psychotherapist, armed with these neurodynamic principles, is thus on the solid neurobiological ground that Freud sought but could not find, and the modern psychotherapy client is spared the indignity, the futility, and the expense of a dream mystique that never did make much sense and is now clearly outdated.

We can summarize all these differences between the two models succinctly. Table 4.1 lists some of the processes involved in dreaming and shows that the explanations offered by psychoanalysis and activation-synthesis are, in almost every case, so different as to force diametrically opposite conclusions regarding the use of dreams in psychotherapy and the means by which that use might (or might not) alter waking consciousness beneficially. It should be obvious that the consequence of changing the dream theory in this way is to force a change in the psychopathological model as well. Before turning to that subject, it will be helpful to discuss some of the contrasts that are apparent in Table 4.1 with respect to their broader implications for psychology. In doing so, I will also indicate some of the sources of error in the psychoanalytic model that arose from the neurobiology used by Freud in the 1890s. This exercise is somewhat technical, but it is important because it highlights a century of progress in our conceptualization of how brain-mind states are generated and how they are altered.

Table 4.1
Two Models Explain the Altered State of Dreaming Differently

Dream Phenomena	Psychoanalysis	Activation-Synthesis
Instigation	Repressed unconscious wish	Brain activation in sleep
Visual imagery	Regression to sensory level	Activation of higher visual centers
Delusional belief	Primary process thinking	Loss of working memory due to DLPFC inactivation
Bizarreness	Disguise of wishes	Hyperassociative synthesis
Emotion	Secondary defensive response of ego	Primary activation of limbic system
Forgetting	Repression	Organic amnesia
Meaning	Actively obscured	Transparent, salient
Interpretation	Needed	Not needed

DLPFC, dorsolateral prefrontal cortex.

Dream Instigation

Because he was so exclusively committed to a reflex model, Freud was unaware of the spontaneous activity of the brain-mind. He could not therefore conceptualize states like dreaming (or the psychosis of mental illness) as the natural outcomes of changes in chemical balance of the brain. No wonder, then, that he regarded dreaming as a universal form of psychopathology. Upon this erroneous view he constructed his entire theory of normal mental life as an intrinsically pathological outcome of compromise between the exigencies of instinctual drive and psychological defense mechanisms. For Freud, dreaming could not possibly arise as the entirely healthy manifestation of emergent consciousness that accompanies normal brain development.

Dream Vision

Freud's psychoanalytic model posited that all of the energy and information in the mind had to come from the outside world. One famous example is that of hunger arising in signals from the body to the brain, which causes the infant who seeks but does not find immediate satisfaction to hallucinate the breast, hence quelling the drive. In Freud's dream and psychotherapy model, every visual image was derived in a similarly secondary, wish-fulfilling way. Freud did not recognize that the visual system was structurally elaborated by genetic program long before birth and that its spontaneous activation in sleep was guaranteed—also long before birth—by entirely intrinsic and spontaneous alterations in brain chemistry.

This is not to say that hungry infants never hallucinate breasts or that hallucinated breasts never serve to stave off sleep-interrupting hunger pangs. Our experience as adults tells us that such mechanisms may sometimes indeed come into play, as when we dream of relieving ourselves in response to sensations arising from a full bladder. But such transformations of bodily or other external stimuli are rare. Most dream stimuli are pseudosensory activation signals arising in the brain stem and relayed to the forebrain for perceptual elaboration. Dream vision is thus a primary perceptual response to phasic activation signals impinging on the thalamus and cortex at what now appear to be high levels of sensorimotor and emotional integration. The view of any and all dream vision as secondary and psychodynamically mediated is an entirely outmoded and indefensible hypothesis. And yet not only do we see no open disavowal of this kind of thinking, we even see it defended by some neuropsychologically sophisticated psychoanalytic apologists.

Dream Delusion

Freud correctly assumed that the failure of self-reflection in dreams that results in our delusional belief that we are awake, can fly, or survive surely deadly falls from vertiginous heights was akin to psychosis. As such we accurately regard it as primary process thinking, which is by definition narcissistic, omnipotent, and uncritical. But why does it have this character? And by what mechanisms? Certainly not to defend consciousness from invasion (because consciousness *is* invaded by primary processes in this case!). It seems far more likely that this failure to test reality is the outcome of an organic deficit related to two other deficit conditions of dreaming, the disorientation that creates bizarreness and the amnesia that creates dream forgetting.

The reason that we are so uncritical, so grandiose, and so uninsightful in dreams is because the working memory guidance system of our dorsolateral prefrontal cortices is disenabled. This defect is very likely to be a function of the embargo that our Dream Drugstore has placed on norepinephrine and serotonin (which become memory, orientation, and judgment pills when we push the drugstore analogy to the limit).

But you might say, hey, wait a minute. Doesn't the construct of an executive system responsible for accurate context assessment, self-reflection, deliberation, and judgment sound just like the ego that Freud said wanted to sleep? Isn't the prefrontal cortex just a stand-in for Freud's ego that kicked off the dream process by relaxing its guard on those unruly id wishes in the unconscious? Sure enough, the deactivation of the dorsolateral prefrontal cortex certainly does rob the dreaming brain-mind of the capacity for such cognitive processes as insight, judgment, and deliberate action. But there is no evidence that the dorsolateral prefrontal cortex "wishes" to sleep or that the shift to hallucinoid, delusional, hyperassociative, and emotion-driven cognition is any way secondary to release of the id from repression. On the contrary, it seems much more likely that the cerebral agencies of both higher order cognition (cortex) and emotion (limbic system) operate in parallel and in reciprocal interaction with the active sleep generating mechanisms of the brain stem.

And these brain stem mechanisms, as we know, have a completely nonconscious mind of their own! It would certainly be presumptuous to suppose that any psychological theory or practice could bring the motives of these low-level but vital structure-function complexes to the light. To say, for example, that the brain stem "wishes" to sleep is to indulge in the most fanciful sort of anthropomorphism. It's like saying that the respiratory oscillator in the medulla is expressing a "death wish" when it stops issuing breathing commands at sleep onset and in REM sleep. But don't let the Freudians get a hold of this one or they will turn it into a first principle that, once again, vindicates the master's prescient insights!

By the way, how would Freud have understood breathing? Certainly not as the expression of an intrinsic brain stem oscillator equipped with its own metabolic energy and its own information encoded in its connections and chemical signals. His model of the brain did not envisage these properties. Using the reflex model he would have to suppose that we breathe in response to external inputs like hypoxia and hypercapnea. Of course the medullary respiratory oscillator is responsive to—and hence driven by—external signals such as blood oxygen and carbon dioxide levels. But its most salient feature, reliable rhythmicity, is intrinsic and has nothing mechanistically to do with environmental vicissitudes. In this sense breathing is just like dreaming. They are both vital, spontaneous, internally prescribed brain rhythms. Moreover, they are dynamically interactive, in that respiration speeds and slows as activation signals from the sleep control system rise and fall. If the signals fall to very low levels, as they do in sleep apnea, the sleep system is switched back to waking to guarantee a resumption of breathing.

Lest you suppose that I am creating a caricature or exaggerating in my representation of psychoanalytic theory, let me remind you that until recently, some patients with narcolepsy, a disease characterized by excessive daytime sleepiness, were treated by psychoanalysts who sought the unconscious conflict motives for their symptoms in early childhood experience using the free association techniques, including dream interpretation! Now, it is certainly true that these patients can benefit from psychotherapy, because their work and social lives are so disrupted by their symptoms. But drugs that neurodynamically enhance waking and suppress REM sleep by boosting the efficacy of the aminergic neuromodulatory systems of the brain stem can immediately reduce the symptoms. Unfortunately, the fundamental defect in narcolepsy antedates even childhood and infancy. It is in the genes! And that is likely to be the case in many of the disabling psychiatric conditions that psychoanalysis has ascribed to interpersonal dynamics early in life.

Dream Bizarreness and Emotion

There are numerous problems with the psychoanalytic concept of dream bizarreness as the product of defensive transformations via disguise-censorship of the unconscious wishes thought to instigate dreaming. First and foremost is the manifest failure of the hypothetical censorship. Dreams, as we have pointed out, are saturated in powerful emotions, many of which have a distinctly raw id-like character: dream elation may be coupled with the most embarrassingly naked narcissistic wishes; dream anger may be associated with decimating murderous rage. But even more problematic for psychoanalytic dream theory is the presence of anxiety, which may reach panic proportions in nightmare dreams.

It is around the model of anxiety that this whole argument turns most sharply. Freud knew that dream anxiety was a problem for his theory. If disguise-censorship was working, what need would the ego have to elaborate defensive anxiety? And if disguise-censorship had failed, why should not all anxious dreams result in awakenings? Freud could not answer either of these questions. But if, as we propose, anxiety, like elation and anger, is simply a primary emotion that we experience when the limbic system is automatically activated in sleep, the problem disappears, and with it goes disguise-censorship and all the rest of psychoanalytic dream theory. Because Freud did not credit the brain-mind with the spontaneity we now know it possesses, and because he could not have known that limbic system activation was intrinsic to sleep, he was forced to hand-wave whenever the question of dream anxiety was raised.

For activation-synthesis, the limbic system is a spontaneous anxiety emitter, as well as reflexive anxiety generator. In this sense, activation-synthesis regards some anxiety, some elation, and some anger as normal and existential, even in waking. Here we border on theories of personality and mood, both of which we can redefine as the mix of baseline emotion that emanates from us as we navigate through our social worlds. This view of anxiety as primary and as natural is extremely liberating. It is also in keeping with the classical Darwinian view of emotional expression as adaptive and communicative. The fact that the three emotion systems mediating anxiety, elation, and anger of the brain-mind are all selectively activated in REM sleep means they can be taken as prima facie evidence of their importance to survival rather than as failures of an imaginary internal psychic defense system.

Positive emotions (called elation, happiness, affection, eros, or joy, depending on the terminology used in their definition) are crucial to approach behaviors, to courtship, and to pair-bonding. Normal people need them in moderation to function well socially. Positive emotion is diminished to crippling degrees in depression and enhanced to crippling degrees in mania. People take street drugs in order to move their moods up. The Dream Drugstore keeps this system working well by running its positive emotion programs off-line at night. In psychotherapy, we should take the presence of elation in dreams as a promising sign that the juices of approach behavior are indeed flowing, not as a sign of weakened dream defenses.

Anger is also adaptive. Before we wound, it warns our predators, be they bullies, rivals, or even intimate encroachers of our boundaries, our territories, and our psychological limits. Anger helps us to define how close or distant we want to be and on what terms! No wonder it is so difficult, even with all the inspiration we can draw from a charismatic leader like the Dalai Lama, ever to rid ourselves completely of anger. (When the Dalai Lama says he loves the Chinese because he always learns something from his enemies, we know we are talking to a master rationalizer and a strategic genius.) And no wonder anger is so prevalent an emotion in dreams. In this view the purpose of dreaming is not to disguise our primitive selves, but to reveal them. If the Dalai Lama experienced no anger even in dreams we would have dramatic proof of the power of positive thinking to cross brain-mind state boundaries. It would also further convince us that mindfulness training should become an integral part of any psychotherapy that wished to reduce anger (or increase joy), simply by providing the waking brain-mind with autosuggestion in the presence of meditation.

Anxiety is a pivotal emotion for clinicians to understand properly because it is so disruptive when it is excessive and because it is so commonly excessive. According to activation-synthesis, it is too much of a good thing rather than a sure sign of childhood abuse. Childhood abuse is real. And trauma is real. And panic anxiety may really be linked to both. But whether anxiety can be relieved via catharsis—by lancing an unconscious boil—is highly dubious. Anxiety can be unlearned. Even though the Chinese don't go away and even though they don't welcome the Dalai Lama back to Tibet, he remains serene in Dharmsala. For the rest of us mortals, anxiety is helpful, up to a point. It is wise to be wary (but crippling to be phobic and psychopathic to be cool to cruelty) and it is useful to be skeptical (but crippling to be paranoid and dangerous to be gullible).

Our dreams link anxiety quite reasonably to the disorientational root of dream bizarreness. We are lost; we have no credentials; we miss trains, boats, or subways; we are improperly dressed; we don't recognize our dream surroundings or our dream companions; and we often do not even know why we are going we know not where! Is each of these anxiety links especially important? I doubt it. Generically speaking, they tell us what we already know, that we live in a social world that is always challenging the adequacy of our preparation and presentation. Mr. Cool, wake up. If you believe you can eliminate anxiety, you are whistling in the dark. Reduce it, yes. To manageable proportions, we hope so. Eliminate it, no. Don't even try. You will become emotionally incompetent.

Dream Forgetting

To suggest that dreams are unremembered because they are re-repressed is illogical and implausible. It is illogical because there is no need to re-press our already disguised wishes. It can't hurt to remember them. So why not remember all of them? It is implausible because there simply is not room in anyone's unconscious to pack all of these dream scenarios (not to mention all the valuable memory capacity that even an incomplete catalog would occupy). Psychoanalysis has underestimated the amount of dreaming because Freud, quite understandably, thought that dreaming occurred only in the instant before awakening. And, indeed, it is probably only those dreams that we *do* remember. That's why awakening studies are so important. They show that we dream at least 90 minutes per night (and probably much more), but at best we recall 5 percent, and that's on a good night. Some perfectly normal people have no recall whatsoever.

Whereas psychoanalysis simply has no means of accounting for the extent of dream forgetting, activation-synthesis can easily and confidently ascribe it to organic amnesia. With the memory molecules norepinephrine and serotonin locked up in the Dream Drugstore and with the working memory circuits of the frontal cortex greatly attenuated, no record of dreaming is ever entered into memory. That's how much stock the brain-mind puts in the content of dreams! It sure looks like we aren't supposed to remember our dreams. That can't be because our consciousness would be damaged by them, as Freud assumed, but it could be because they contain useless or even misleading information that is better ignored than taken too seriously. As psychotherapists we ought therefore to be wary of focusing too much attention on them.

Using the Neurodynamics of Dreaming in Psychotherapy

I myself enjoy having dreams and I enjoy discussing them with friends, colleagues, and family members—especially my wife. It doesn't seem to do any harm; nor can I say it does any particular good. But as a talking point it is certainly more interesting than the weather or most of the news, and sometimes it even rises to the level of a great film or a novel. This is because of the obvious emotional salience of dreams and because, like great works of literature, they are about us.

This is essentially the same position I take with my psychotherapy patients and my psychotherapist students. I try to convince both groups that dreams are unusual mental products that teach us volumes about the normal workings of the mind and that contain all of the seeds of abnormality within them. Because dreams are so psychotic they put me and my most deranged patients on the same playing field. By thinking about my dreams—and theirs—I can more easily imagine what it is like to be psychotic when awake.

I can appreciate how completely taken over my perceptions could be were I to hallucinate. I understand, on contemplating my delusional lack of insight when dreaming, how unwelcome and futile it would be to try to talk me out of a paranoid belief. Because when dreaming I believe the most bizarre dream events are real, I know that weirdness is no sure tip-off that I am out of my mind. And, more importantly, I can use the experience of dream hallucination and delusion to create an alliance by directly (sometimes) and indirectly (always) communicating my understanding of the power and subjective reality of psychosis.

In taking this tack, I am careful not to trivialize or patronize. Having hallucinations while awake is considerably more frightening and debilitating than while asleep. This is obvious, but this too I know from first-hand experience. Fortunately, all of my experience of waking psychosis has been circumstantial and easily understandable. Sleep deprivation is one sure way to get psychotic, and closed head injury is another. I've had both. But I dream almost every night and so am constantly reminded of the thin line that separates "us" from "them." It is so thin as to suggest that except for the vicissitudes of our brain-mind states "we" are all "them." But because I can use the autosuggestion method to prime my brain-mind later to pick up my dream madness—precisely because it is so bizarre—I can begin to teach my students and patients to use cognitive tricks to monitor their own states and to alter them in desired directions. Lucid dreaming thus informs lucid waking—by which I mean knowing that I am crazy when I am crazy by curing myself when I am sane. If I know I am crazy, it at least gives me the chance to control my madness by using more cognitive tricks.

One of my schizophrenic patients helped me understand this quite clearly when she told me that she could stop her visual hallucinations simply by counting the ceiling tiles in her bedroom. How could this work? By directing her eye movements voluntarily and by focusing her attention on a specific part of the visual world, and by using her cognitive apparatus to actively analyze and compute features of that world, she was able to tip the balance of power between internal (hence dreamlike) image generation and the external image generation of normal waking.

Before she was on antipsychotic medication and after she stopped taking her pills she couldn't do this at all. So I could also use her self-correcting talent to reinforce the need to maintain adequate levels of medication and even to explain, in a rough way, how blocking her dopamine receptors helped to damp out her psychosis. In the later section on the Medical Drugstore, I will come back to this point. For now, suffice to say that the fact that I can control my own dream psychosis by becoming lucid or by waking up tells me, my patients, and my students that tipping the chemical balance in the brain is the key to successful therapy, be it psycho- or pharmaco- or both!

I have learned other tricks from my own memory problems and those of my patient informants. First and foremost, I know just how totally helpless one becomes when recent memory fails. Dreams emphasize this point through the frequency of these disconcerting, incomplete arrangement scenarios that we have already considered. Without recent memory I am lost, disoriented, feel confused, get very anxious, and run around in circles. So armed with dream neurodynamics, I can empathize more effectively with amnesics, and I can advocate a gamut of remedies more authoritatively.

One remedy is self-priming. As I have gotten older and more forgetful, I have learned to take more time and more trouble "reminding" myself. Another remedy is to uncouple the anxiety from the amnesia (because I see how voraciously they feed on each other in my dreams). Instead of becoming angry or anxious when I can't recall a name, I cognitively steer my amygdala into safe harbor and either ask unembarassedly for help, or wait long enough for my weakened memory search engine to find the data. It often works!

The negative feedback reciprocity between anxiety and effective memory search is classic. The psychodynamically inclined call it blocking— as if the memory failure were due to repression. This concept is so deeply engrained that I dare say there is not one reader of these words who has not at some time declared, "I'm blocking on that" and meant that your amnesia was an example of the overdetermined psychopathology of every day life—you blocked because of unconscious conflict.

An alternative explanation is that you simply couldn't immediately locate your identifier data, felt embarrassed on that account, then got anxious, and next fell into the vicious cycle of pre-emption of the search engine by the anxiety. But look, amnesia is quite common. You have it every night in your dreams. And it makes your anxiety worse, right? If, as we have seen, that process is not caused by conflict but by competition between brain regions, its waking equivalent might be more easily accepted and understood. The take-home message here is that the wisdom of age is simply learning to do more with less. It's a strategic matter; you don't want to wipe out the capacity of what little cognitive capability you still have by succumbing to panic, do you? No. You want to keep your bearings and give the search enough time to succeed.

The Use of Psychedelic Drugs in Psychotherapy

Not everyone can remember dreams, and many of the dreams that we remember are banal. Dreaming may thus be too weak a phenomenon to allow anyone to appreciate the direct and indirect didactic impact of dreaming. The realization that sanity and insanity are separated by a fine line and that insanity has its own instructive form may be lost on many of us.

Why not, then, resort to stronger medicine? Why not use substances like LSD, which can reliably alter consciousness in striking and memorable ways? This rationale is enormously strengthened by the claim that drug-induced states are genuinely transcendent. That is, they not only instruct us about hidden aspects of the natural world, but they open our eyes to other worlds that are qualitatively unique.

In the drug culture of the midcentury many people were easily persuaded by these arguments. In their book *Psychedelic Drugs Reconsidered,* Lester Grinspoon and James Bakalar point out that there were more than 1,000 clinical papers describing psychedelic drug test results with over 40,000 patients published between 1950 and 1965. LSD was used in the treatment of psychosomatic and neurotic disorders, schizophrenia and autism, the rehabilitation of criminals, alcoholism, and even the pain of dying. Elegiac testimonials extolled the virtues of LSD treatment in tones that are more typical of hyperbolic autosuggestion and religious conversion than of sober self-reflection. As an example of hyperbolic autosuggestion, one woman wrote that after four years of psychoanalysis, 23 LSD trips had not only convinced her of the validity of Freud's theories, but cured her of her symptoms as well:

I found that in addition to being, consciously, a loving mother and a respectable citizen, I was also unconsciously, a murderess, a pervert, a cannibal, a sadist, and a masochist. In the wake of these dreadful discoveries, I lost my fear of dentists, the clicking in my neck and throat, the arm tensions, and my dislike of clocks ticking in the bedroom. I also achieved transcendent sexual fulfillment. . . .

At the end of nine sessions, over a period of nine weeks, I was cured of my hitherto incurable frigidity. And at the end of five months, I felt that I had been completely reconstituted as a human being. I have continued to feel that way ever since. (Grinspoon and Bakalar, 1997, p. 198)

As an example of religious conversion we turn to the famous Hollywood actor, Cary Grant, who showed that he could be as histrionic off-stage as on when he ascribed nothing less than rebirth to his 100 LSD sessions:

The first thing that happens is you don't want to look at what you are. Then the light breaks through; to use the cliché, you are enlightened. I discovered that I had created my own pattern, and I had to be responsible for it . . . I went through rebirth. The experience was just like being born for the first time; I imagined all the blood and urine, and I emerged with the flush of birth. (Grinspoon and Bakalar, pp. 198–199)

Despite these extravagant claims, there were no well-controlled studies that could have evaluated them scientifically—and the possibility of doing any such studies was quashed by law. Whether we should regret or celebrate this forced shut down of inquiry is open to debate. The conservative in us says good riddance to bad rubbish. The liberal in us is horrified by any form of governmental suppression of inquiry.

From the safe distance of 25 years we can perhaps obviate the political aspect by examining the two major assumptions on which all of this work was based. I will argue that both are certainly problematical and probably completely unfounded.

The first assumption was that by taking psychedelic drugs, subjects were rendered less depressed, anxious, guilty, and angry, and more self-accepting, tolerant, deeply religious, and sensually alert. In other words, subjects were not only made more amenable to psychotherapy, but were actually transformed in the same desirable directions that therapy would take them.

The second assumption was that the drugs could help induce the powerful experiences of regression, abreaction, intense transference, and symbolic drama that were the process goals of psychodynamic psychotherapy.

These assumptions illustrate the two major fallacies of the psychoanalytic era: the failure to control for placebo effect (against which psychotherapy of any kind has difficulty competing), and the adherence to the cathartic model of psychoanalysis (which assumes that you can only get better if you get worse).

Armed with our new vision of dreaming and the techniques for accessing, entering into, and even directing them, it would seem that we have, at least, an alternative to pill-popping and to mind-blowing. There is no clear evidence that psychedelic chemicals do any permanent harm, but there are certainly risks of acute derangement, errors of judgment, and behavioral excess that one might later regret. Dreaming, by contrast, can be equally wild, but it is guaranteed to be completely safe as long as we don't project our delusional hopes on it. Because it is also legal—and free—it satisfies both the puritanical and the parsimonious aspects of our character at the same time as it turns our limbic system loose from the reins of restrictive reason.

5

The Neurodynamics of Dissociation, Hypnosis, and Autosuggestion

If we are allergic, phobic, or just reasonably cautious about taking drugs, what can we do to alter our own states of consciousness in psychologically desirable directions? How does the relaxation response take place? What is the mechanism by which meditation achieves its salubrious effects? What, in neurobiological terms, is the power of positive thinking? And even if I am not capable of entering into a deep trance or turning hallucinations on and off at will, how can I use hypnotic techniques to achieve such mundane but practical consequences as reducing the pains of dentistry, childbirth, or cancer?

Before taking up these—and other fascinating topics like lucid dreaming—it is important to recognize that they all partake of a process called dissociation. Dissociation is the hybridization of one set of state features with those of another. It has traditionally been seen as pathological—as in Jean Martin Charcot's famous cases of hysteria who could not, for example, perceive pain or speak, although they were apparently conscious and the physiological systems mediating the impaired functions were intact. But dissociation can also be regarded as a natural propensity of normal brain-mind states, as modern sleep and dream science amply demonstrate. Moreover, as with Charcot's cases, the natural propensity for dissociation can be facilitated or primed via deliberate interventions of an accomplice (e.g., a hypnotist, a therapist, or a bed partner) or by one's self.

All that we need to get on with the show is to develop a general model of dissociation and to create a do-it-yourself kit for the induction of desirable dissociations. In this view, Charcot's hysterical anesthesia becomes our way of cutting out the anesthetist and the novocaine injection.

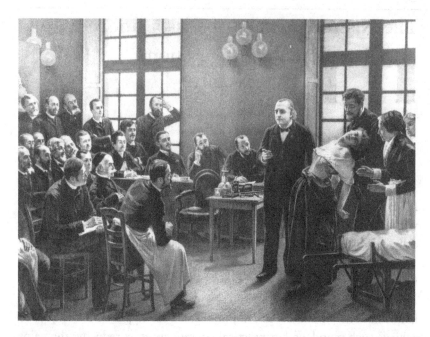

Figure 5.1
The French neurologist Jean Martin Charcot (1825–1893) was famous in his time in part because of his dramatic demonstrations and bold interpretations of the altered states of consciousness and behavior that he induced by using hypnotic suggestion with his patients at the Salpêtriere Hospital in Paris. Because his patients' complaints could not be explained by existing neurological knowledge, he opened the door to the invention of psychoanalysis by Sigmund Freud, who received a fellowship to study with Charcot and was impressed with his mentor's emphasis on the sexual conflicts of his patients as unconscious causes of their symptoms. Charcot and Freud were unaware of the nervous system's inherent propensity to change its own state in a manner that favored the dissociations that fascinated them. (Detail from painting by Andre Brouillet. Reproduced courtesy of the Anna Freud Museum)

Although Charcot (figure 5.1) and Sigmund Freud are well known as the champions of psychogenic dissociation mechanisms, the French psychiatrist Pierre Janet (figure 5.2) must be credited with the most detailed and critical scholarly treatments of this subject. It was Janet, for example, who recognized the similarities between the alterations of consciousness in sleep and hypnosis (see also table 5.1, figure 5.3). In fact, he coined the term *somnambulism* (whose literal meaning is sleepwalking) to describe hypnotic trance. Of course, none of these theorists

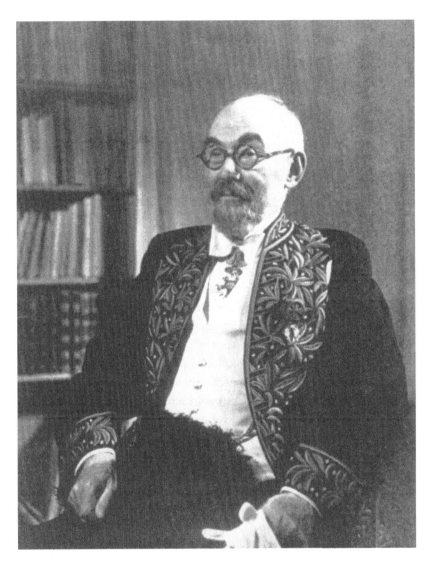

Figure 5.2
Pierre Janet (1859–1947) was a psychologist who shared Charcot's interest in those dissociative phenomena that arose spontaneously and could be hynotically induced in patients, especially those females who were called hysterics. Janet's emphasis was upon personality structure, which could be conceived of as an integration of conscious and unconscious ideas and tendencies. He thought hysteria was due to a lowering of psychic activation, which (as in sleep) resulted in varying degrees of dissociation. Like William James, Janet was encyclopedic in his learning and versatile in his interests; he wrote many papers and books but never formulated a brain-based theory of association and dissociation. (Reprinted by permission of the Archives of the History of American Psychology, The University of Akron)

knew enough about the brain to formulate a physiological theory of dissociation.

What Is Dissociation?

Dissociation is the separation of modules of consciousness that are usually associated with one another. A good example is the usual association of perception and movement with memory and conscious awareness. In post-hypnotic suggestion, the subject executes a command for which there is no conscious recollection. The subject clearly perceived the command (witness its execution), but cannot remember having been given the command.

Dissociation is a robust phenomenon with dramatic and specific clinical meaning, but it has until now been without any secure tie to underlying brain activity. As an initial attempt to formulate a brain model of dissociation, it may therefore be strategically useful to examine some far less dramatic and even commonplace dissociations that occur at the boundaries of major states of consciousness. Many of these dissociative phenomena already have known physiological substrates, and others may constitute more reasonable targets for neurobiological analysis than clinical dissociations.

Examples of dissociations of consciousness that often divide the waking mind into two compartments include microsleeps, attentional lapses, and fantasy states. At the edges of sleep are hypnagogic hallucinations and sleep paralysis. Within sleep are sleep walking, sleep talking, and lucid dreaming. In all of these conditions, consciousness has some features characteristic of one state mixed with features characteristic of another.

Dissociations at the Level of the Brain

Consciousness is currently best conceived as the brain's awareness of its own activity, including such modular functions as perception, memory, thinking, and feeling, each of which has some degree of anatomical localization or functional specialization with which to begin model building. It follows that for conscious states to be fully *associated*—that is, characterized by a unified and internally consistent set of properties— the several anatomical and physiological substrates of each of the several component modules must be perfectly synchronized and perfectly integrated.

The easiest way to appreciate how *dissociation* might arise neurobiologically may be to consider the "split brain" as both a paradigm and a metaphor. When subjects have their corpus callosum cut, each of their two half brains is conscious but neither can be fully conscious of the other. This kind of split-brain is a literal and concrete dissociation: there are two states of consciousness coexisting independently in the same brain. The two states of consciousness are not complete: one half of the brain (usually the right) can perceive normally but not verbalize its conscious experience because language is (usually) on the left.

More subtle, functional cleavages occur, and it is these that can be instructive as we attempt to understand the neuropathology of dissociation, for example, divisions between our cognitive and emotional response to an individual. Where the concrete example is horizontal (the split brain in the midline), most functional splits are vertical (the split brain between higher and lower brain regions).

Another way to look at the brain in terms of association-dissociation is to consider the task of unifying and integrating neuronal ensembles. Given the known vastness and complexity of the brain as a colony of neurons, how is unity, harmony, and synchrony possible? Recent estimates place the number of elements at 100 billion, and although most of the cells involved in consciousness are probably in the head, it is still critical to tie forebrain activity to that of the spinal cord, a distance of about one meter.

If any subcolony of cells were to become unruly—read hyperexcited— what would happen to the rest? They would either go about their business (setting up the prospect of unconscious dissociation) or deal with the rebellious colony in some way akin to civil war, opening up the prospect of conscious dissociation.

Epilepsy is an extreme case of neuronal rebellion and illustrates a spectrum of functional dissociative possibilities. In *grand mal* there is marked takeover and chaos; in *petit mal* there are lapses; in temporal seizures there are fugues, automatisms, and elaborate, long-lasting subdivisions of consciousness.

The Fallible Substrates of Association

Multiple interconnectivity (each cell simply contacting, say, ten thousand others) must help reduce the chances of neuronal schism and secession. But this is not enough. Some multiply connected cells are chemically specialized so as to produce uniform microclimates in far-flung and remote corners of the neuronal empire. Although many of these systems overlap, they are not 100 percent redundant, which means that chemical microclimates may differ radically at different brain latitudes and longitudes. Examples include the *noradrenergic locus coeruleus* and the *serotonergic raphé complex,* both of which send widely ramifying axons up and down the neuraxis from the strategic and central location in the brain stem (see figures 2.3, 2.4).

These two systems appear to operate in spatial parallelism and in temporal harmony. Although there are important differences in both the cortical sections and layers within sectors to which they project, there is also extensive overlap. Their strong interconnection at the level of the brain stem may well contribute to their temporal synchrony with the outputs of both cell groups being strongly correlated to the level of arousal and to receptivity to external stimuli.

Despite the safeguards of redundancy and strong coupling, the very fact that there are two such systems provides a potential substrate for dissociation. As yet, no evidence for spontaneous dissociation of the two systems has been reported, but pharmacological interventions that selectively weaken or strengthen one system are abundant, and these are often associated with dissociative symptoms (e.g., amnesia), impulsive behavior in keeping with the character of the affected individual, and feelings of depersonalization and derealization. All of these findings suggest that neuromodulatory neuronal systems, normally thought of as mediators of associative process (e.g., attention, alertness, memory) may, when altered, mediate dissociation.

In this view, the unities of consciousness and of personality are seen as the result of dynamically negotiated balance, coordination, and cooperativity between populations of neurons.

The Battle of the Mind—Competition Between Neuromodulatory Systems

The normally harmonious music of the aminergic neuronal spheres is contrapuntal to the brain stem cholinergic system, whose modulatory output is generally reciprocal to the aminergic groups and distinctly phasic and burstlike in character (rather than tonic and regular). In fact, the phasic bursts of acetylcholine (ACh) neuronal discharge appear to be strictly and precisely related to eye movement control by the paramedian reticular formation and the oculomotor system.

This means that extreme eye movements (as in upward eye rolling and gaze fixation) could produce powerful changes in cholinergic output. Because we know that the activation of this system is a hallmark of REM sleep and because REM sleep is fraught with dissociative phenomena (e.g., amnesia, hallucinations, bizarre mentation, anxiety, and loss of volitional control), we take further interest in some of the properties of this unique neuronal population. Do highly hypnotizable people have inherited or learned hypersensitivity of the cholinergic system such that shifts to a dreamlike state are precipitated directly out of waking?

Some features of the cholinergic system are germane to this question. Rather than projecting directly and diffusely to forebrain sectors, the brainstem cholinergic projections are both more limited in distance and more precisely targeted—they project to the ipsilateral thalamus and sub thalamus. From the basal forebrain, other cholinergic neurons project to the cortex.

These features are compatible with a role in the feedforward integration of eye movement commands (and perhaps other brain stem motor outputs such as gait) but also in the feedback control of thalamocortical sector activation. No such function has previously been suggested, but the intimate connection of eye movement variability, volitional change (frontal eye field), and sensorimotor facilitation and blocking warrants serious consideration of this hypothesis.

Regional Reciprocity and Dissociation

Complementing the balance between aminergic dominance (with exteroceptive focus, linear thinking, and rationality) and cholinergic dominance (with interoceptive focus, analogical thinking, and emotionality) is the recently demonstrated shift in blood flow from the dorsolateral prefrontal cortex (the seat of working memory, directed, analytical thought, and related executive systems) to subcortical limbic structures like the amygdala and parahippocampal cortex (the seat of emotion-driven unconsciousness, instinctual processing) during REM sleep.

What we call intuition is, in fact, the tuning in of emotion-based unconscious processing and the tuning out of logical operations. "I *know* he's a really nice guy, but I get a queasy gut feeling that tells me he's dangerous!" Gut feelings are so named because they are the metaphor and the conscious experience of involuntary autonomic nervous system activation like stomach churning, rapid heart action, and sweating that are automatically triggered by the limbic system when a stimulus generates fear and anxiety.

In some therapeutic settings we may want to decondition the stimulus if it has been overlearned or generalized from truly traumatic experiences in the past to truly innocent experiences in the present. In order for that to happen it is important to relax one's guard strategically (via the relaxation response or nitrous oxide inhalation) so that relearning can take place. Such interventions, which are commonly used in behavior therapy, dampen aminergic and simultaneously enhance cholinergic neuromodulation. This not only allows the emotional response to occur safely and tolerably, but also to dissociate it from its overgeneralized past stimulus and to reassociate with more modern and specific contexts.

Another way to appreciate the regional contributions to dissociation is to consider the feeling we call "spaciness" when our dorsolateral prefrontal cortex relinquishes its hold on our consciousness and we lose contact with our environment. This loss may become a gain, however, if we want to deliberately enhance emotion-driven cognition as in fantasy, literary imagining, or dynamic psychotherapy. By having patients lie on a couch and say whatever comes to mind, Freud was trying to get the dorsolateral prefrontal cortex out of his office and to give full rein to his patients' amygdalae! His interest in dreams stemmed from the same motive, even if he didn't know the mechanism underlying the shift from what he called secondary to primary process thinking.

Making the unconscious conscious is, after all, the boldest dissociative goal imaginable. And if Freud could boast of his successful self-analysis, why can't we? Even if we don't follow his metapsychological assumptions, we can still enjoy looking at our dreams for what they tell us about our emotional impulses, as well as for their intrinsically powerful scenario structures.

Lucid Dreaming

When I just said "looking at our dreams," I meant, of course, reviewing our recollection of dreams as they may be remembered after the fact. For many of us, this is the best that we can do. And, sadly enough, some of us can't even do that. But the phrase "looking at our dreams" really means dissociating a part of our brain-mind that can "look at" the operation of the rest of "our dreams." In other words, we want one part of our brain-mind to be awake enough to watch and another part to be asleep enough to continue to dream. This rare but learnable talent is usually called lucid dreaming and is most economically defined as the bolstering of the self-reflective awareness that is normally diminished or absent in dreaming.

What can sleep neurophysiology and the new neuropsychology tell us about lucid dreaming, and how can we use that information to increase our access to that state? And what, beyond entertainment, can we learn about the brain-mind from a scientific exploration of lucid dreaming? The last question has one ready answer: by placing experienced lucid dreamers in a PET scanner (or preferably an fMRI), we could test the hypothesis that, when lucid, dreamers increase the blood flow to their dorsolateral prefrontal cortices as that cortex reactivates to a level consistent with wake state executive function.

In order for the dream to continue (so that it can be observed), the pontine activation would have to persist, and with it, all the outward signs of REM sleep (including the inhibition of muscle tone and the REMs themselves), as Stephen LaBerge observed in his laboratory studies of lucid dream adepts. We would also predict that the amygdala activation would decline reciprocal to the dorsolateral prefrontal increase and with that decline, negative emotionality, especially fear, might also diminish.

Indeed, it is an empirical fact that lucid dreamers experience less negative emotion and more positive emotion in their altered states of dreaming! Some therapists even use the inculcation of lucidity to tame negative dream affect. This can become an effective treatment for nightmares that is to be preferred to pharmacology (which has side effects) and to long-term psychotherapy that may neither uncover nor quell the hypothetical traumatic nightmare stimulus. The dreamer simply says to the fear, "Hey look, this is my dream, get out and let me enjoy it!" Sounds good, doesn't it? And it is. But how easy is it to accomplish?

Science and Psychedelics

The reason that I enjoy lucid dreaming is both scientific and psychedelic. When I first heard about the possibility—from my hostess at a Kennedy-era Washington dinner party—I was trying to learn about hypnosis, which, following Freud's injunctions, had been banned from the psychiatric curriculum at the Massachusetts Mental Health Center. I had just witnessed operative dentistry under hypnotic anesthesia with my colleague Bob Drury, so I was open to the possibility that suggestion could alter dream consciousness without the use of external chemicals. At that time many of my colleagues, including my NIH boss Ed Evarts, were experimenting with LSD. I didn't mind giving it to animals to see what it did to REM sleep, but I didn't want to take it myself because I was apprehensive about becoming psychotic (on the spot) and experiencing after effects (years later).

My dinner party hostess, who happened to be a descendent of Mary Arnold-Foster, sent me home with her copy of *Studies in Dreams,* where the technique of lucid dreaming and its psychedelic delights are described in detail. I was as attracted by the idea of flying in my dreams as I was by the power of self-hypnosis, so I followed Arnold-Foster's prescription. I simply put a notebook by my bedside, so as to be able to record my dream recall, and told myself, before going to sleep, I'll pay attention to my consciousness, which I would know to be dreaming because of the bizarre discontinuities and incongruities of time, place, and person.

My response to this simple autosuggestion technique was typically three-tiered. First, I became much more aware of dreaming. Within a week I was flooded with more recall than I could record. Second, I was progressively more aware that I was dreaming while I was dreaming. At first this was simply a supposition, like "this is too weird to be waking reality, I wonder if I'm dreaming." Then this doubt gave way to the conviction that, yes, this is a dream, and I'm watching it happen. Third, I became able to exert volitional control. This control could alter an ongoing plot like changing my movement from running to flying, interrupt the dream (so that I could briefly awaken, secure recall, and then return to the dream), or initiate a preordained plot (such as to induce the perception of brightly colored kaleidoscope-like imagery that was completely abstract).

After a couple of weeks of practice I was flying hither and yon, meeting important people (like JFK!), and making love to all manner of oneiric bed partners in the safety and privacy of my bedroom and my dreams. The positive emotions—giddy elation, surprise, delight, humor, and erotic excitement—were all there in great abundance, even if they sometimes gave way to fear, anxiety, and doubt as non-lucid dreaming regained the upper hand.

These self-observation experiments convinced me of the veracity of lucid dreaming as a robust and remarkable state of dissociated consciousness. What other conclusions can we draw from the experience of lucid dreaming?

First (and foremost for this book), we can alter consciousness voluntarily and without the use of drugs to achieve many of the formal desiderata of the drug-induced psychedelic states. These include the simulation of psychosis, with exotic visual imagery; the simulation of magical behaviors worthy of Carlos Casteneda's imaginary Don Juan; the cultivation of ecstatic elation; and the experience of highly erotic sexual adventures. What else is there? Well, you might say, what about religious transports? Unification with the Godhead? "Why not?" I reply. If that's what you want, you can probably get it, as did Emmanuel Swedenborg, whose induction procedure included intentional sleep deprivation to potentiate the REM process on which lucid dreaming rides. I'm not religious, but I bet I could hallucinate angels, saints, or even the Trinity if I tried!

Second, it clearly demonstrates that we can master simple, safe, and economical self-hypnosis techniques. This observation has broad implications for psychiatry, for medicine, and for human behavior generally. That a voluntary practice can influence even so highly automatic and instinctual a state as REM sleep dreaming means that faith can indeed move mountains (physiological mountains, that is). This, of course, is a knife that cuts both ways. We can either be enlightened or fooled by such evidence, depending upon the theory we are testing. It would seem to me as erroneous, for example, to conclude that my faith in God was experimentally validated by seeing him in my dreams, or to conclude that because I could fly in dreams I could with impunity awake and jump off the Empire State Building's observation deck.

Third, it shows that a kind of psychic causality—or free will if you will—operates in conjunction with brain physiology. This last point illuminates the others and is so important as to deserve critical analysis. In the section that follows I consider the possible brain basis of lucid dreaming and develop a cognitive neuroscience theory applicable to all dissociative states where suggestion plays an important part.

The Brain Basis of Lucid Dreaming

In order for me to escape total absorption in my dream I must somehow be able to dissociate some part of my brain-mind from REM sleep so that it—the dissociated part—remains awake or regains the waking state while the rest of my brain-mind dreams on. I must, therefore, do nothing less than change brain physiology and chemistry, at least locally, by the medium of thought. Sounds spooky, doesn't it? No wonder so many hard-headed scientists reject the reality of lucid dreaming!

But I think that the explanation may be quite straightforward. All we need to do is cobble together several well-established cognitive science building blocks and then do a crucial experiment.

The first building block is the robust memory mechanism called priming. We know that a word—and if a word why not a sentence—can prime subsequent recall so that associated words are more easily recognized. And we know that sleep, especially REM, may even enhance this priming, especially for weak primes. The explanation offered for priming is that the neuronal networks underlying associated words are activated by the prime word (or sentence).

It is this sort of mechanism that I think must underlie the incubation procedure for lucid dreaming. By putting the notebook at my bedside and by telling myself to be on the lookout for dream bizarreness, I am actively priming my mnemonic neural networks with instructions whose activation may be strong enough to persist or to reactivate when REM sleep supervenes. Enough of each activation in a localized part of my brain might then be able to resist co-option by the REM sleep activation process that would normally take over or eliminate its influence.

Where might such neural networks reside? In the cerebral cortex for sure, and in the dorsolateral prefrontal cortex for odds on bets. Why? Because that's where working memory resides, and we're talking about working memory when we want to notice what is going on, analyze it, and make executive decisions based on our analysis. Another very compelling reason for zeroing in on the dorsolateral prefrontal cortex is that it is one of the only cortical regions that is selectively deactivated in REM sleep, an observation that fits perfectly with the usual impoverishment of working memory, self-reflective awareness, and executive functions like volition in REM sleep dreams.

Now we need to tie the priming with its residual activation of dorsolateral prefrontal cortex neuronal networks to the emergence, in REM, of a reactivation of those networks. I propose that the residual activation of the dorsolateral prefrontal cortex is amplified by the REM activation of these other cortical networks that produce dream bizarreness via the associative resonance that the dorsolateral prefrontal cortex has been primed to detect. And indeed, the dawning awareness that "this must be a dream" feels, subjectively, like a positive feedback process. Once the recognition has been inserted into delusional process it is enhanced by the mounting evidence of delusion that it observes!

At this point, a delicate and tenuous balance is in place between delusion and insight. The lucid dreamer must now be careful to let the delusional process run wild enough to give a good ride but not to run away from (at least) observation or (at most) control. Tip the balance too strongly in favor of insight and we wake up. Tip it too strongly in the direction of delusion and we lose lucidity!

It is as if we were designed to be rational (but cool) and irrational (but hot) by turns. How difficult it is, at all times, and in all states, to maintain the balance between reason and emotion. Among the subcortical systems that we suppose might be less powerfully activated during lucid dreaming are the amygdala and (perhaps) the parahippocampal cortex. To maintain the hallucinatory intensity of the dream we would expect the pons and the parieto-occipital junction cortex to remain activated.

The predictions of an experiment to test this hypothesis are thus clear. The subjects are available and the scanning technology is in place. Why hasn't the experiment been done? Because it hasn't yet been proposed. Why not? One reason is that many more descriptive experiments need to be done first; a second is that no serious neurobiological research has ever been done on lucid dreaming. A third reason is that this is high-risk, expensive work. PET scans are single snapshots, yielding instantaneous cross sections of brain perfusion. Lucidity is a rare and evanescent phenomenon, as seemingly evanescent today as dreaming was in 1950! So we may have to wait a while before this study can be done. I hope I am alive—and awake—to see it.

Hypnotic Trance and REM Sleep Dreaming

If it is possible for us while awake to implant the suggestion that we should later, in sleep, notice that we are dreaming, it is quite easy to imagine that someone else, a hypnotist for example, could implant in us while in trance the suggestion that we perform some specific act when we later awakened. Because it may not be easy for many of us to imagine going into a trance at all, the analogy that I will now develop between hypnosis, dreaming, and lucid dreaming may be particularly instructive. In essence the analogy depends upon the similar interplay, in both hypnosis and dreaming, of the factors shown in table 5.1. In studying the table and in reading the following discussion it is important to realize that hypnosis is *not* sleep. Rather it is a dissociated state of waking into which many of the features of sleep have been inserted. In this sense it is the precise reciprocal of lucid dreaming, where some features of waking have been inserted into sleep.

Sensory Aspects
When a subject enters the hypnotic state, awareness of the outside world diminishes, just as it does at sleep onset. Reciprocal to this diminished

Table 5.1
Parallel Interplay of Phenomenological Factors in Hypnosis and Dreaming

	Hypnosis	Dreaming
Responsiveness to external stimuli	Diminished (in light trance) to anesthesia (in deep trance)	Diminished (in sleep onset dreaming) to hypoanesthesia (in REM dreams)
Hallucination	Enhanced in deep trance	Enhanced in sleep onset dreams to markedly enhanced in REM sleep dreams
Movement	Disfacilitated to paralyzed in deep trance	Disfacilitated to paralyzed in REM dreams
Orientation	Sometimes impaired	Poor for times, places, and person
Volition	Voluntarily suspended	Diminished (at sleep onset) Lost in REM sleep
Memory	Amnesia for state; enhanced memory for remote events	Amnesia for state; enhanced memory for remote events

acuity to external stimuli is an enhancement of internal awareness in both sleep and hypnosis. In the case of sleep, this enhanced internal awareness may proceed directly to hallucinosis, whereas in hypnosis hallucinosis occurs only in deep stages of trance. It is significant that in hypnosis subjects can maintain communicative contact with their surroundings even in deep trance, when they may experience anesthesia; this is virtually impossible in dreaming, which is similarly anesthetic. In lucid dreaming, however, subjects who awaken to their state do not suddenly become fully able to converse with their environs but can signal out—by a coded set of voluntary eye movements—their awareness that they are dreaming.

What this means is that the threshold to external stimuli is raised and lowered at will within waking (in hypnosis) and involuntarily within sleep (in dreaming). Whether the threshold adjustment is voluntary or involuntary, there tends to be a reciprocal enhancement of internal sensory stimuli that reaches hallucinatory strength easily (in dreaming) and with more difficulty (in trance). This particular feature of hypnosis strengthens the claim that hallucination, the most severe and stigmatic symptom of mental illness, can be triggered in two entirely natural states. Hallucination is thus a normal propensity of the brain-mind, whose emergence is a function of natural changes in brain-mind state.

Motoric Aspects and Volition

The facilitation of entry into hypnosis by muscle relaxation and immobility is mirrored by sleep onset. Control of the motor system must be abandoned by subjects wishing to abet either process. This at first passive deactivation of the motor system can proceed to frank paralysis in the deepest stages of trance and emergent REM sleep when the active inhibition of motor output is instantiated. The suppression of movement in deep hypnotic trance appears to be caused by extreme defacilitation of motor networks rather than active inhibition, and hence it can be overcome by strong stimulation and strong effort.

Needing emphasis is that voluntary movement is difficult or impossible in both REM sleep dreams and deep trance. It is this feature—the loss of volition—that may be a deeply unifying factor, even if it is caused by quite different mechanisms. In any case, the threshold to movement, like the threshold to external sensation, can be voluntarily or involuntarily raised so that immobility is guaranteed. But this does not mean that movement cannot be simulated, imagined, and perceived as real. It can. And it is perceived, with spectacular verisimilitude, in both states.

So now we know that both sensation and movement mechanisms evince the same external dampening and internal stimulus release in both states. We therefore can't help wondering if the same kinds of neural processes underlie these strikingly parallel and reciprocal phenomena.

Orientation and Memory

Amnesia is a cardinal feature of hypnotic trance and dreaming. Dreamers upon awakening and hypnotic subjects emerging from trance may have great difficulty or be completely unable to recall their experience. In the case of hypnosis there can be no doubt of the amnesia because the subjects cannot recall behaviors that were outwardly observable. In the case of dreaming, the presence of equally vivid but virtual behaviors can be safely inferred from the results of REM sleep awakening studies that yield reports of highly animated and florid movement scenarios that would otherwise have been completely forgotten.

Because recent memory is disenabled in both states, it is not surprising that orientation to time, place, and person is impaired in hypnotic trance and dreaming. That this process is considerably more floridly deranged in dreaming may possibly be due to the more extreme changes in neuro-modulatory balance that occur in REM sleep (for details see subsequent discussion).

The general rule that every loss entails a gain applies to memory as well as to sensation. Just as hallucinatory capacity rises and exterocep-tive sensibility declines, so does access to remote memory increase as recent memory capacity declines. Thus dreams are subject to invasion by characters and situations from the long-lost past and hypnotic subjects may find their way to memories of early experiences that are germane to self-understanding. A caveat, in both cases, is the obvious susceptibil-ity of both states—but especially hypnosis—to the suggestion of false or factitious memory. So far, no one has attempted to use the hyper-amnesia of dreaming as a lens for sleuthing recovered memory. So far, so good!

Common Processes Suggest Common Mechanisms

If hypnosis and sleep are not identical, how might we understand their shared propensities in the cardinal domains of sensation, movement, voli-tion, and memory? Put another way, how might the conspicuous dissocia-tions shared by the two similar but distinct states be mediated in the brain? To address these questions we will recur to the three-dimensional AIM model and show that hypnosis and lucid dreaming converge on the same region of the state space (figure 5.3). Hypnosis moves subjects down toward the forbidden zone at what we might call the upper limits of REM sleep. The reason that the two states do not converge is because the mech-anisms by which the system achieves its start points (wake vs. REM) are quite different, even if the processes that move them away from these start points are quite similar. Let me explain.

To move from wake to deep trance, subjects must deactivate the cortex, especially the dorsolateral prefrontal cortex; the same structure must be reactivated to move from non-lucid to lucid REM dreaming. The deacti-vation, in the case of hypnosis, facilitates the loss of contact with the outside world, the abandonment of the will, and the amnesia while

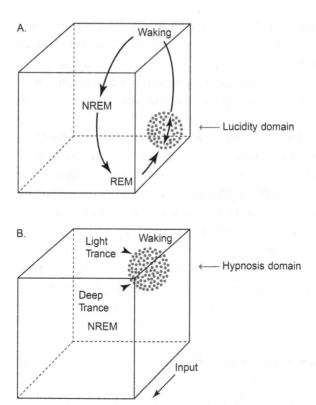

Figure 5.3
(A) Lucid dreaming. When subjects become aware that they are dreaming they have regained some aspects of waking consciousness while retaining aspects of REM sleep. The lucid dreaming domain is thus uneasily poised between REM and waking. Lucid dreaming is an unstable state and there is a strong tendency to either wake up or return to REM and thus lose either the dream or the lucidity. (B) Hypnosis. In hypnosis, activation may decline or shift regionally as subjects focus on internal information and exclude external inputs. An obvious limitation of AIM is exposed in this example. It cannot reflect the changes in regional activation level which are documented in neuroimaging studies.

allowing the reciprocal upsurge in hallucinatory and emotionally salient remote memory from the limbic and paralimbic regions. It is these very qualities, naturally maximized in REM, that need to be diminished to allow the dreamer to increase self-reflective awareness, reinstate volition, and dampen negative emotion.

The upshot is that hypnosis and lucid dreaming both result from oppositely directed changes in the balance of regional activation levels that drive AIM toward a forbidden zone with congruent but reciprocal phenomenological features.

These reciprocal movements in AIM state space involve simultaneous and reciprocal changes in input-output (I) and modulatory (M) balance, as well as altering the balance of regional activation.

Internal inputs are enhanced in hypnotic trance and suppressed in lucid dreaming, whereas aminergic drive is suppressed in hypnotic trance but enhanced in lucid dreaming.

These decreases in the I function occur in trance because external stimulus strength declines. We now note that the opposite movement of the I function in lucidity is the reciprocal enhancement of inputs external to the REM system, but rather than coming from the outside world, they come from the primed dorsolateral prefrontal cortex, which has been instructed to notice—and act on—dream bizarreness by dissociating itself from REM.

Now we need also to note that the cholinergic system moves toward convergence as it is (a) suppressed from its peak in REM as lucidity develops and (b) released from its inhibitory suppression in waking as trance develops. These oppositely directed changes in neuromodulatory balance (trance = less aminergic, more cholinergic; lucid dreaming = more aminergic, less cholinergic) may actually be causally related to the regional activation shifts via the influence of the neuromodulators on regional blood flow and they may contribute to the shift in input-output balance via their regulatory role on the subcortical phasic activation systems that we can describe under the rubric of PGO waves. As discussed in greater detail in chapter 7, PGO waves are the EEG signs of internally generated signals from the visuomotor system, which generates REM in the brain stem, to the visual sensory and perceptual structures of the thalamus and cortex. To enhance lucidity we need to tune the PGO waves down (more aminergic, less cholinergic), whereas to enhance trances we need to turn them on (less aminergic, more cholinergic).

Neuroimaging of Hypnosis, Meditation, and Dreaming

Recent neuroimaging studies of altered waking states such as meditation and hypnosis shed light on the similarities and differences between such states and dreaming. They have shown that, even in waking, enhanced activity of posterior areas of the cortex that subserve rich internally generated somatosensory experiences such as visual imagery can occur when frontal cortical executive controls are weakened, as they are in dreaming.

In a recent Danish PET study of yoga mediatation, Hans Lou and colleagues remark on the similarity of this state's brain activation pattern to that of REM. The absence of anterior cingulate activation in meditation is attributed to the emotionally bland character of the meditation performed compared to the emotional turmoil of dreaming.

Pierre Maquet of the University of Liege in Belgium has recently reported that hypnotized subjects show increased activation of posterior (sensory experiential) cortices with no corresponding increase in frontal (logical, "executive") areas. The degree of self-motivated involvement in the meditation practice seems to strongly affect the activation status of these frontal areas. This fact was revealed by a recent fMRI collaboration between the Behavioral Medicine and Neuroimaging groups at Harvard, who showed that meditators repeating a self-generated mantra to achieve the relaxation response activated frontal attentional systems. They thought this might be as a result of the attentional effort involved by their particular technique.

The result of all this new work is that an objective comparative neurophysiology of altered states of consciousness is in the making. As the technology of brain imaging continues to improve and the number of studies using this exciting approach grows, it will become more and more important to characterize the conscious experience, the motivation, and the intentions of the experimental subjects. No amount of expensive gadgetry can make up for heterogeneous and ill-documented subjectivity. For that reason, we conclude this chapter with one historic account of trance that illustrates the utility of the expert witness paradigm of conscious state research.

Aldous Huxley's Deep Reflection

Good descriptions of trance states are hard to come by. Because the very name "trance" has such spookily provocative connotations we are not tempted to learn about it. One consequence is that those of us who are not easily able to enter such altered states tend to be ignorant of what it actually feels like. We may even be fearful of the implied loss of control. The upshot is a tendency to discount the whole story as a fabrication, so we can remain safely and smugly skeptical. But if we continue to ignore trance, we miss the opportunity to learn from it and to better understand it.

Aldous Huxley's (figure 5.4) capacity to enter—at will—the dissociated state he called "deep reflection" is of value because Huxley was a painstaking self-observer. Anyone who cut his novelistic teeth (as I did) on such brilliant books as *Antic Hay* or *Point Counter Point* will share my admiration of Huxley's wit, his literary elegance, and above all, his interest in interpersonal relationships. He is a very special kind of expert witness to his own unusual states of consciousness, which he actively cultivated in the service of his writing. Because Huxley's interest in the vicissitudes of altered states extended to mysticism and to psychedelic drugs, he is an ideal contributor to our inquiry into the Dream Drugstore. One final point: Huxley was so open that he was willing to collaborate with the hypnosis expert Milton Erickson (figure 5.5), despite having his own biases. Erickson's involvement provides a valuable and welcome degree of objectivity.

Erickson met Huxley in his Los Angeles house in 1950, and they spent the day experimenting together and making extensive notes. Because Huxley's own notes were lost in the tragic brush fire that later destroyed his home and library, we rely on Erickson's for a description of Huxley's deep reflection as a state

marked by physical relaxation with bowed head and closed eyes, a profound progressive psychological withdrawal from externalities but without any actual loss of physical realities nor any amnesias or loss of orientation, a "setting aside" of everything not pertinent and then a state of complete mental absorption in matters of interest to him. Yet, in that state of complete withdrawal and mental absorption, Huxley stated that he was free to pick up a fresh pencil to replace a dulled one to make "automatically" notations on his thoughts and to do all this without a recognizable realization on his part of what physical act he was

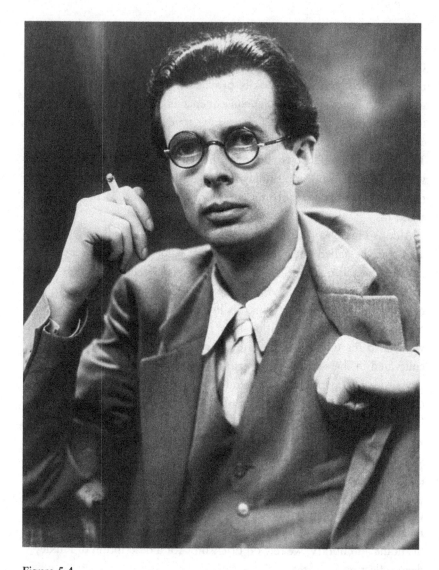

Figure 5.4
The British author Aldous Huxley (1894–1963) was the grandson of Thomas
Henry Huxley, commonly known as Darwin's Bulldog. But instead of champi-
oning science, as did so many of the Huxleys, Aldous used his far-ranging intelli-
gence, his graceful style, and his mocking humor to create a series of novels
conveying contrasting ideas and opinions and then to explore philosophy and
mysticism. With the publication of *The Doors of Perception* in 1954, Aldous
Huxley became an early exponent of drug-induced alterations of conscious states,
a position he maintained and expounded upon toward the end of his life, as he
lost his own visual capacity and the psychedelic movement embraced him warmly.
(Photo © Bettmann/Corbis)

performing. It was as if the physical act were "not an integral part of my thinking." In no way did such physical activity seem to impinge upon, to slow, or to impede the train of thought so exclusively occupying my interest. It is associated but completely peripheral activity. . . . I might say activity barely contiguous to the periphery. (p. 47 in Tart, 1969)

Huxley was able to enter his state of deep reflection in about five minutes. He simply "cast aside all anchors" of any type of awareness and thereby achieved an "orderly mental arrangement" that permitted his thoughts to flow freely as he wrote. When he demonstrated this, Erickson observed that Huxley was completely out of touch with his surroundings, a feature that was amply confirmed by Huxley's wife, who often found him sitting in his chair oblivious to the world while his behavior was "automatic like a machine moving precisely and accurately." It took him about two minutes to emerge, after which he described the "timeless, spaceless void" that he had left, and "a total absence of everything on the way there and on the way back and an expected meaningless something for which one awaits in a state of Nirvana since there is nothing more to do."

Huxley could alter the features of the state by autosuggestion or upon Erickson's instruction. He could see color or he could limit his descent to a lighter level and still retain contact with Erickson. But like subjects in the forbidden zone of lucid dreaming, Huxley tended to be pulled deeper or to exit when his concentration was interrupted by verbal or nonverbal commands. In other words, the introduction of volition, presumably mediated by the frontal cortex, acted in opposition to the trance state.

When he tried to induce auditory and visual hallucinations, Huxley found it difficult to remain in trance unless he built up the hallucinatory scenario by attaching the sound of music to the sense of rhythmic body movement. When Huxley moved the music up to the level of opera so that he could hear singing, he was observed by Erickson to be mumbling.

This constructive process, by which motor commands become the internal stimuli for sensory experience, is exactly what occurs in REM sleep dreaming when oculomotor and vestibular signals generate dream imagery. When this process was going on inside Huxley's head, Erickson observed changes in Huxley's head position and in his breathing pattern.

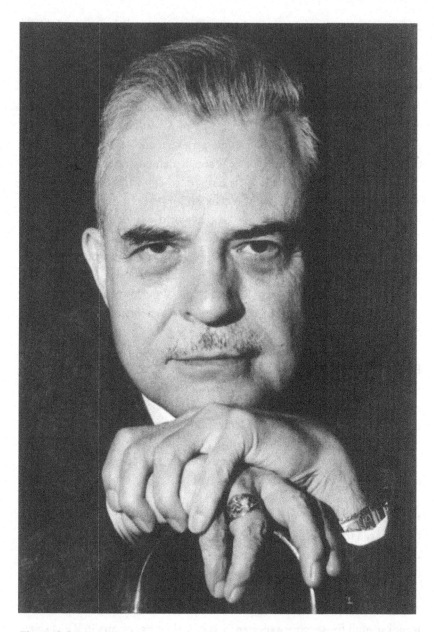

Figure 5.5
The psychoanalytic movement was at pains to suppress and distance itself from hypnosis because Freud wanted to be sure that his patients' revelations and the benefits he supposed would result from their uncovering were not the product of

By feeling his head turn from side to side Huxley was able to evolve a giant rose, three feet in diameter, from what was at first a barely visible rhythmically moving object.

Several other formal features of Huxley's trance condition are of interest with respect to the analogy we have drawn with REM sleep dreaming. We first consider the relaxed posture, indicating a step on the path to cataplexy. In full-blown cataplexy, the assumption of a flaccid posture is associated with the inability to move on command and is thus similar to the active motor paralysis of REM sleep dreams. Anesthesia and amnesia were both present in Huxley's trance, although they tended to be selective, and when Huxley attempted to make them global, his trance deepened. Time distortion, a distinctive component of the orientational instability of dreams, was a robust aspect of Huxley's altered state.

A most dramatic finding was Huxley's ability, in 65 percent of the trials, to give the correct page number when passages of his books were read to him. Huxley claimed that he could recall most of his writings at will, so that when he heard a passage he could then mentally read the antecedent and subsequent paragraphs, whereupon the page number "flashed" into his mind. This almost incredible feat of hypermnesia is paralleled in dreaming by the unbidden emergence of characters and incidents from the distant past; it contrasts, significantly, with the loss of recent memory capacity. It is as if the loss of the diminished capacity to record were complemented by or compensated for by an enhanced capacity to play back! The mechanism of this reciprocity must be explained both at the level of regional circuitry and at the level of neuromodulatory balance.

Even more incredible is the description of age regression, the final tour de force of the Erickson-Huxley encounter. I give a passage to convey

suggestions. The American psychiatrist Milton H. Erickson (1902–1980) was among those who resisted Freud's injunction because he thought that hypnosis could be used effectively both for diagnostic exploration of the unconscious and for effecting desired changes in behavior. Now hypnosis—and related practices like relaxation and meditation—are becoming more widely accepted and lending themselves to scientific study to determine their underlying brain mechanisms. (Reprinted by permission of the Milton H. Erickson Foundation, Inc.)

the claim directly and to let the reader decide what to make of it:

He turned back and noted that the infant was growing before his eyes, was creep-
ing, sitting, standing, toddling, walking, playing, talking. In utter fascination he
watched this growing child, sensed its subjective experiences of learning, of wanting, of feeling. He followed it in distorted time through a multitude of experiences
as it passed from infancy to childhood to school days to early youth to teenage.
He watched the child's physical development, sensed its physical and subjective
mental experiences, sympathized with it, empathized with it, thought and wondered and learned with it. He felt as one with it, as if it were he himself, and he
continued to watch it until finally he realized that he had watched that infant
grow to the maturity of 23 years. He stepped closer to see what the young man
was looking at, and suddenly realized that the young man was Aldous Huxley
himself, and that this Aldous Huxley was looking at another Aldous Huxley,
obviously in his early fifties, just across the vestibule in which they both were
standing; and that he, aged 52, was looking at himself, Aldous, aged 23. Then
Aldous, aged 23 and Aldous aged 52, apparently realized simultaneously that
they were looking at each other and the curious questions at once arose in the
mind of each of them. For one the question was, "Is that my idea of what I'll be
like when I am 52?" and, "Is that really the way I appeared when I was 23?"
Each was aware of the question in the other's mind. Each found the question of
"Extraordinarily fascinating interest" and each tried to determine which was the
"actual reality" and which was the "mere subjective experience outwardly projected in hallucinatory form." (p. 66 in Tart, 1969)

The question of whether such experiences are "actual reality" or "mere
subjective experience outwardly projected in hallucinatory form" is
central to current debate that pits "veridical experience" against "false
memory" and pits multiple personality against role-playing. Although
Huxley's apparently exceptional ability to enhance recall by altering the
state of his brain and our own ability in dreams to relive early experience
are clear evidence that memory is state dependent and can be altered,
none of the evidence supports the now thoroughly discredited idea that
every experience, thought, and feeling is recorded in the brain-mind forever and is therefore theoretically retrievable. And none of it counters the
strong positive empirical evidence that memory is easily distorted or even
fabricated in response to social demands.

What hypnosis now needs to advance as a science is the application of
the scientific principles and techniques that other Huxleys developed,
from Thomas Henry Huxley (1825–1895), who championed the theory
of evolution as "Darwin's Bulldog," to Andrew Fielding Huxley (1917–),
who advanced the ionic hypothesis of the nerve action potential and won

the 1963 Nobel Prize for Physiology and Medicine, and Hugh Ensor Huxley (1924–), whose sliding filament theory of muscle contraction explained how chemical energy is converted to movement.

How, we wonder, would a PET scan of Aldous Huxley's brain in deep reflection compare with the images collected in outwardly attentive waking, deep sleep, and that most easily obtained altered state of consciousness, REM sleep dreaming? My guess is that it would look more like REM than deep sleep or waking.

Part III
Normal and Abnormal Alterations of Consciousness

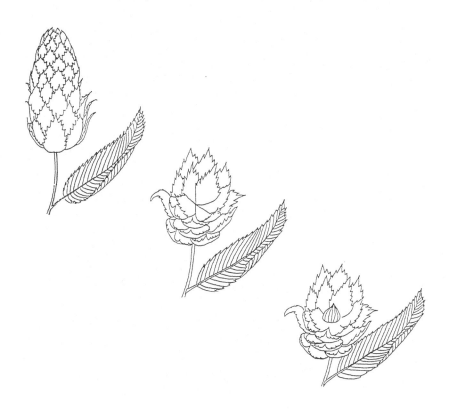

6
The Brain-Mind and Its Conscious States

I define consciousness as subjective awareness of the world, the body, and the self. This definition includes awareness of awareness but, because it does not depend on it, allows for the occurrence of the kind of consciousness that occurs in dreaming. In dreaming, the world that we are aware of is entirely fabricated, but we do not know it. Only when we awaken and regain awareness of awareness—and with it insightful perspective—do we know that we were previously deluded.

Allowing for partial, differentiated, and even delusional states of consciousness is not only accurate but also strategic. It is strategic because it allows us to compare states of consciousness missing one or another feature of consciousness with states when that feature is present. This strategy—which I call *phenomenological subtraction*—lends itself nicely to the cognitive neuroscience enterprise. In fact, it maps perfectly into the strategy of subtraction used in modern brain imaging studies like those I alluded to in the last chapter when I tentatively ascribed the subtraction of self-reflective awareness from waking consciousness to the subtraction of the full functionality of the dorsolateral prefrontal cortex in REM sleep.

Measuring Consciousness

Consciousness has been off limits to science for almost a century because subjective experience was thought not to be objectifiable. Although I understand why positivist critics of mentation are worried about this issue, I think it is fundamentally mistaken. Furthermore, I think the problem can be solved and, more shockingly, I am sure that it has been solved! Before you close the book or even snicker condescendingly, please hear me out. How can I be sure, you ask skeptically, that all of those dreams that I reported in chapters 2 and 3 really occurred? And how can I be sure that, if they really occurred, they really occurred before I woke up and "remembered" them? Couldn't they have occurred as part of the awakening process and then been erroneously back-projected into sleep?

If I assert that my memory, however impaired by age, is still quite good, and add that I am a highly overtrained observer, you will quite correctly chide me with hubris because you know that personal recollection is notoriously unreliable. Two people who have seen the same crime or alleged criminals often can't agree on the details well enough to convince a jury of what they saw.

In the case of consciousness, you say, the situation is even worse because, by definition, no one else can see my dreams but me. And I would agree with that. I don't ask you to consider the details of my reports as scientific evidence, and I don't ask you to take my interpretation of those details as scientific proof of any particular dream theory.

All I ask is that you look with me at the thousands of reports of dreaming that have been accumulated by scientists around the world and analyze their formal properties as I do. By formal properties I mean such general properties of conscious experience as sensory modality (does the report contain a description of vivid vision and of movement?), coherence (does the report have internal consistency, or is it highly discontinuous and incongruous?), emotional quality (was the affect neutral, or was it charged, especially negatively?) and so on, through questions about self-reflection and directed thought and memory.

If there were consensus on all of these matters—and there is—you would have, at least, to concede that half of the objectivity battle—that of reliability and with it face validity—was won. Otherwise you would be forced to hypothesize that the consensus about formal properties was illusory and that the subjects (including me!) were just making up stories to satisfy expectations. This argument invites a reductio ad absurdum rejection. What motive could possibly be satisfied in this way? And how could all of the subjects know what was expected of them, as the very notion of formal properties is recent and the specification of them an ongoing project? Many people don't even understand what the term means when it is explained to them.

Naturally, dream content is likely to be extremely variable from subject to subject, gender to gender, age group to age group, and culture to culture. But the formal properties—like visual imagery, bizarre sequencing, and poor memory—are more likely to be universal because they are biologically based. Using formal properties as a measure, observations about dreaming are at least as reliable as scale readings by laboratory technicians.

What about the validity of dreams? Do they really pertain to mental activity, occurring in real time, during sleep? Here again, the answer is convincingly, consistently affirmative. It has been repeatedly observed that the longest, most vivid, most bizarre, and most affectively charged reports are offered following instrumental (or spontaneous) awakenings from REM sleep. Further, all of these formal properties have increased intensity when the REM sleep preceding the report was physiologically intense. What else do we need to know? Well, maybe, you skeptically suggest, all of those correlations are valid but simply predict that a convincing dream report will be constructed during the awakening process.

Although it is difficult to label dreams with external stimuli (because the brain in REM sleep actively excludes them), it can, with persistence, be done. When a bell is rung or the skin is tickled, subjects often incorporate the stimulus properties into the ongoing dream scenario. This temporal labeling of dreams with external stimuli clinches the point. I hesitate to add the evidence of lucid dreaming, because for many of my colleagues it is controversial and unconvincing. But I am convinced by it, in part because I have personally confirmed the experience of lucidity, and in part because I find Stephan LaBerge's data to be persuasive (even if I don't subscribe to many of his interpretations and extrapolations of the data).

If I begin with my reservations, I might be better able to disarm the critics. If I am able to regain awareness of awareness in my dreams and so know that I am dreaming, I am not in a statistically normal state of dream consciousness. From this it follows that I cannot have such an experience in statistically normal REM sleep. So I disagree with LaBerge and others of his school when they assert that lucidity is less exceptional than I suppose and that it requires no special alterations of REM sleep. This is an important point for reasons that will become clear later in this chapter.

So what impresses me about the LaBerge data? The fact that his sleep lab subjects can motorically signal out, from ongoing dreams, that they are dreaming, and have the dreams continue, and voluntarily change the plots of those dreams. I have done it all myself, though not in a sleep lab and not without self-awakening. But so what? I can become aware that I am dreaming, prove that I am veridically and voluntarily dream conscious by waking myself up, and prove that dreams occur in real time by voluntarily returning to sleep, recognizing dreaming, and voluntarily altering the plot!

All an illusion, you say? That was a false awakening that didn't really occur. You have no objective evidence of it. "Rubbish!" I reply. "You are again forced back to the wall of absurdity. I know I (sometimes) have false awakenings (from REM) and I know what they are like, just as I know I sometimes have confusional, confabulatory awakenings (from NREM) and I know what they are like. These problematical exceptions must be acknowledged and they must be explained, but they must not be allowed to confound signal and noise (or baby and bath water)."

The main reason for accepting my subjective judgment of these experiences is that in laboratory studies they correlate with physiology. In false awakenings, the subjects are in fact still in REM sleep, whereas in confused, confabulatory awakenings, they are, instead, in NREM sleep. Both of these conditions illustrate dissociation perfectly. In false awakening, I dream that I woke up (and fulfilled my obligation to the experimental protocol!), whereas in confusional arousals, I really did wake up enough to deliver a report while parts of my brain were still deeply asleep.

The fact of the matter is that by accepting all of the safeguards that the skeptic rightly demands and rejecting only the most absurd alternative hypothesis, we can confidently conclude that consciousness can be objective about itself. How else could consciousness be functionally adaptive and why else would it be evolutionarily conserved?

State Carry-Over Paradigm

When we awaken from REM with vivid dream recall, we *carry over* the subjective experience of dreaming into subsequent waking. But is that all there is to it? Do we not, perhaps, carry over some of the physiology, too? How complete, and how instantaneous, is our conversion from REM to wake? We would almost certainly be wrong if our awakenings were complete (100 percent) and instantaneous (0 latency). But exactly how long does it take us to change state, and what exactly are the processes that delay the transition?

Sleep inertia is an easily understood concept and an easily demonstrated phenomenon, especially on awakening from NREM sleep, when it may take 15 minutes or longer to shake the lethargic hangover that so powerfully pulls us back down to our beds. There it is clear from EEG recordings that the inertia is in the brain synchronizing process itself (or in the metabolic processes underlying brain activation). Figure 6.1 demonstrates the periodic ebb and flow of brain activation in sleep. Parts A and B emphasize the NREM-REM fluctuations that occur every 90 to 100 minutes, and part C shows that each REM sleep activation phase is accompanied by increases in the level of many physiological functions throughout the brain and body.

When the relay elements of the thalamocortical system are maximally deactivated (in stage IV NREM sleep) early in the night, our ability to regain alert waking consciousness is severely impaired. Sleep lab awakenings performed at this time may even be impossible if the criterion for waking is showing a fully desynchronized EEG and cognitive competence. Slow waves may persist in the EEG of subjects who struggle with confusion and disorientation as they try to give accounts of their subjective experience or perform cognitive tasks. In these cases, which are made worse by sleep deprivation, we can objectively demonstrate subjective accounts to be unreliable, and so should discount them or treat them with great skepticism. That's the bad news.

The good news is that because this strong sleep inertia can drag elements of the preceding sleep stage into waking, it is possible to measure those elements by performing cognitive tasks and/or assessing brain activity directly (e.g., with fMRI). The cognitive neuroscience of sleep depends on such studies because it is impossible for subjects to perform behavioral tasks while fully asleep.

Cognitive Science and Sleep

I should point out that most cognitive tasks measure unconscious mental processes, not conscious ones, so there is still no substitute for introspection if the cognitive neuroscience of consciousness itself is our goal. But

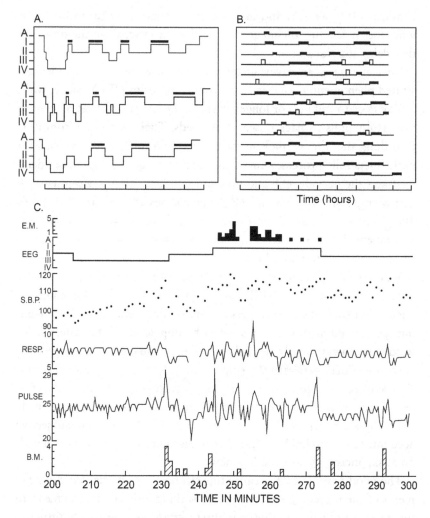

Figure 6.1

Sleep cycle with periodic activation. (A, B) Ultradian sleep cycle of NREM and REM sleep shown in detailed sleep-stage graphs of 3 human subjects (A) and REM sleep periodograms of 15 human subjects (B). In polysomnograms of (A), note typical preponderance of deepest stages (III and IV) of NREM sleep in the first two or three cycles of night; REM sleep is correspondingly brief (subjects 1 and 2) or even aborted (subject 3). During the last two cycles of night, NREM is restricted to lighter stage (II), and REM periods occupy proportionally more of the time with individual episodes often exceeding 60 min (all 3 subjects). Same tendency to increase REM sleep duration is seen in (B). In these records, all of which began at sleep onset, not clock time, note variable latency to onset of first (usually short) REM sleep epoch. Thereafter inter-REM period length is relatively we can use cognitive tests to get at important building blocks of consciousness like memory and perception, either (1) by taking advantage of the state-carry over effect, or (2) by waiting until that effect is over (or both). In the first case, we focus on the cognitive neuroscience of sleep itself, and in the second, upon the functional consequences of sleep for subsequent cognition. Two examples illustrate these approaches.

Sleep Alters Associative Memory Processes

Dreaming has been thought to be hyperassociative ever since 1804, when David Hartley first suggested that we dream in order to loosen connections in associative memory and thus to prevent the obsessive persistence of over-learning. In Francis Crick's modern translation of Hartley's principle, we dream in order to forget. Whatever its function, it is clear that the phenomenon of loose associations in dreaming is germane to understanding dream bizarreness. This is because the incongruities and discontinuities that constitute dream bizarreness clearly demonstrate looser associative processing.

Incongruities such as the dream character who has the physical attributes of one person that we know and the face of another illustrate an indiscriminate but perhaps functionally significant over-inclusiveness in the categories of unconscious memory systems. We can get at this process by using semantic memory tests of subjects awakened from REM and tested both immediately and later when the sleep inertia is over. Compared to waking and to NREM sleep, we find the expected REM enhancement of weak primes (i.e., loose associations) but, to our surprise, not of strong primes (strong associations).

The result is a valuable research tool in itself that we can now use as a probe for, say, the effects of drugs on associative processing in sleep. But it is also valuable because it objectively validates inferences made entirely on the basis of introspective reports. This closes the circle of doubt on introspection and encourages us to proceed, albeit cautiously, in our quest for the neural and chemical underpinnings of conscious experience.

constant. For both (A) and (B) time is in hours. (F. Snyder and J. A. Hobson, unpublished observations). (C) Eye movements (EM), EEG, systolic blood pressure (SBP), respiration (resp), pulse, and body movements (BM) in a 100-min sample of uninterrupted sleep over successive minutes of typical sleep cycle. Entire interval from minute 242 to 273 is considered to be REM period, even though eye movements (heavy bars) are not continuous. (From Hobson, 1998)

Sleep Enhances Learning

If we want, instead, to know if the alterations of consciousness we are assessing in sleep are beneficial or not, we can use cognitive tests to measure learning before and after sleep. Two kinds of learning can be assessed: semantic (which involves words and language) and procedural (which does not). In this case, it is expedient to focus on a non-linguistic task, visual discrimination, which subserves procedural rather than semantic memory. Visual discrimination learning is highly sensitive to subsequent sleep, as Robert Stickgold has recently shown.

Subjects who show *both* robust early night NREM sleep and late night REM not only retain but actually improve their ability to detect a visual pattern accurately and quickly when retested the next day. I should emphasize that this is *not* sleep learning in the usual sense of the word—putting a tape recording of a French language lesson under your pillow and playing it all night is not likely to find you either well rested or fluent in French the next day! But it may mean that more basic skills—and perhaps even French speaking—that are practiced during the day time are actively elaborated and advanced during subsequent sleep.

With respect to drug-altered states, the question naturally arises: do drugs that are typically used to enhance sleep affect sleep learning? We already know some of them affect sleep cognition. For example, the serotonin reuptake blockers can result in the subjective experience of continuous dreaming, an effect on consciousness that may correspond to the drug's ability to enhance rapid eye movements, causing them to occur all night long while, at the same time, blocking REM sleep itself. These drugs cause two kinds of dissociation: first, the eye movements are no longer so strongly confined to sleep with EEG activation; and second, dreaming becomes continuous. Our new cognitive tools, together with our Nightcap and our quantitative dream probes, will enable us to answer these kinds of questions in the near future.

Conscious State Mediation in the Brain

It is already clear from the forgoing discussion that the brain must be fully activated to process information efficiently. Brain activation may have quite different cellular and molecular mechanisms and a quite different regional distribution according to whether it is activated in waking or in REM sleep. The consequences for conscious experience may be correspondingly different in the two states.

The Thalamocortical System

In both waking and dreaming, consciousness depends on the physiological condition of the upper brain. More specifically, the brain stem must continually activate the billions of brain cells that constitute the cerebral cortex and thalamus if we are to be fully aware (waking) or even partially so (dreaming). Here is how thalamocortical activation is brought about.

When the thalamocortical system is left to its own devices, it naturally produces neuronal oscillations which the EEG reads out as spindles and slow waves. These internal reverberations prevent the processing of external signals (as in waking) or of internal signals (as in dreaming) that contribute to the distinctive conscious experiences of these states. In both brain-activated states, the cerebral cortex and thalamus are influenced by signals from the lower brain stem that stabilize their reciprocal circuits by preventing the intrinsic oscillations at EEG spindle and slow wave frequencies. These signals, which include powerful modulatory inputs from the pontomesencephalic cholinergic neurons and the (probably) glutamatergic paramedian reticular formation, depolarize the cells of the thalamic reticular nucleus. These, in turn, project inhibitory GABAergic messages to the thalamocortical oscillatory cells. Cortical GABAergic cells may also dampen the intrinsic thalamocortical oscillations. The net effect is to arrest the burst silence mode of firing of these cells that seem to be the very essence of NREM sleep.

Of course, the absence of consciousness in deep NREM sleep and the weaker dreamlike consciousness of light NREM sleep does not mean that information is not being processed. In fact, evidence is mounting to suggest that the brain may be iteratively processing its recent inputs in NREM sleep as it (perhaps) transfers data from the hippocampus, where it has been temporarily stored, to the cortex, where it can be distributed and filed appropriately for longer term use.

Here again we see that subjective experience is a relatively weak but still informative source of mechanistic and functional insight. Consider the case of sleep following excessive—and therefore novel—daytime experiences like deep sea fishing (for landlubbers) and downhill skiing (for urban couch potatoes and office-bound bunnies). The bed seems to keep moving and the legs keep churning until deep sleep wipes out our awareness of our brain's interactive replay of its unfamiliar inputs. Too much studying can have the same, perhaps useful, effect on the brains of students—overlearning. Cramming may result in all-night reiterations that prevent good sleep but keep the data fresh in short-term stores for regurgitation into blue books the next morning. But, in this case, it may be the blue books—and not the students' brains—that keeps the learned data over the long term! Without good sleep, it may be impossible to incorporate the learned information into a permanent repertoire.

I should also emphasize that NREM stages I–IV occupy 75–80 percent of the time spent asleep, and that NREM is phylogenetically older than REM. These facts witness NREM's evolutionary conservatism and continuing functional importance—even if we remain quite ignorant and perhaps unfairly uninterested in it. Put another way, should we not more actively celebrate NREM sleep as nature's most powerful way of altering consciousness—by obliterating it? From the psychedelic point of view, NREM sleep may seem like no trip at all. But it is certainly not a *bad* trip, and I myself find its transports utterly beguiling. The descent into mental oblivion that I welcome each night has its own special sensuality that I liken to the good meal and to the lovemaking that hasten its advent. And, of course, it ushers me into the natural psychedelic theater of my REM sleep dreams.

The Brain Stem and Conscious State Differentiation

So far, we have mostly emphasized the role of activation in raising or lowering the probability that the brain-mind will be more or less conscious. The electrophysiological evidence of a centrencephalic activating system is echoed by data from recent imaging studies that show that as our mental lights go out, the blood flow to these same core structures declines dramatically.

In addition to the cholinergic and glutaminergic reticular neurons already described as ebbing and flowing in concert with the rest of the centrencephalic core, the brain stem also contains the important aminergic nuclei, the locus coeruleus (secreting norepinephrine) and the raphé (secreting serotonin). We are now moving into the chemical domain measured as factor M in the AIM model. Because the locus coeruleus and raphé neurons have the greatest range of activity across the wake/NREM/REM sequence, we place great emphasis on the possible contribution of their modulatory (M) effects on the different modes of consciousness associated with brain activation in waking and in REM sleep.

These two neuronal groups are of capital importance to our story for two related reasons. The first is that although they appear to modulate the activated forebrain so as to facilitate the distinctive functions of waking (such as attention, perception, linear logical thinking, and recent memory formation), they appear reciprocally to demodulate these same activated structures in REM sleep so as to facilitate the distinctive features of dreaming (such as visuomotor hallucinosis, bizarre imagery, hyperassociative cognition, and emotional storm).

The second is that it is precisely these two aminergic systems (and with them the dopamine-acetylcholine modulatory forces) that are most sensitive to manipulation (for better or worse) by psychoactive drugs, be they prescribed by licensed doctors or sold by street merchant outlaws.

The reasons for ascribing these crucial conscious state differentiating functions to the brain stem aminergic neurons are robust and multiple. The first and most unexpected fact is that whereas the aminergic neurons reduce their firing rate and neurotransmitter release by about half in NREM sleep, they arrest firing completely and stop releasing neurotransmitters almost entirely during REM. This means that aminergic neuromodulation has a quasi-linear—or at least highly quantitative positive relationship—to waking consciousness and a negative relationship to dreaming consciousness. They can thus explain what activation alone cannot: the *differences* between waking and dreaming. Activation can explain only the similarities.

The second and not at all unexpected fact is that drugs that interfere with the release, reuptake, or receptivity to these agents alter consciousness in an informative variety of dreamlike directions. Because this is the central thesis of this book and the one that distinguishes this book from its predecessors, I will elaborate it in detail as we proceed.

For now, simply recall the LSD-serotonin connection and the amphetamine-dopamine-norepinephrine connection: the former causes instantaneously dreamlike waking as it blocks serotonergic neuromodulation; the latter causes delayed dreamlike waking as the inhibited REM process slips away from its suppressers in sleep and breaks through into waking. In both cases the result is, of course, a kind of psychosis.

The Dorsolateral Prefrontal Cortex

The activated cerebral cortex is differentiated not only chemically by the state dependent release of aminergic and cholinergic neuromodulators, but also locally via the interplay of cortico-thalamic, cortico-cortical, and cortico-limbic circuits. These three systems appear to govern, respectively: (1) the sector of the outside world to which we pay attention (via input channel selection by the thalamocortical system); (2) the relative strength of instinctual and emotional forces mediating fight-or-flight survival serving reflexes (via the eruption of anxiety and aggression from the limbic lobe); and (3) the moment-to-moment review of priorities for evaluation and action (via working memory and motor initiative in the dorsolateral prefrontal cortex).

In this hierarchical scheme, the dorsolateral prefrontal cortex is a head ganglion for deliberate decision making, an arbiter and executor of conscious processing, and a director of what we call our will. No doubt oversimplified and minimizing for heuristic purposes what must be constant and massively parallel interactions with other parts of the system, this model is particularly attractive in the context of our conscious state paradigm.

The dorsolateral prefrontal area is a cortical region that shows consistent and conspicuous deactivation during REM sleep compared to waking. Other areas (vide infra) are *more* active, but the dorsolateral prefrontal cortex is less active. What might this observation mean at the level of mechanism and function?

I will address the mechanistic implications in the following section on cortico-limbic interaction. With respect to function, the most immediate and compelling hypothesis is that the subtraction of the dorsolateral prefrontal cortex from the otherwise highly activated forebrain maps on to the subtraction from waking consciousness of self-reflective awareness (self-evaluation), lack of capacity to direct thought (active evaluation), and failure to enact deliberate behaviors, however fictive, in dreaming consciousness (volition).

Add to this mix the conspicuous failure of recent memory to keep dream data in mind for more than a very few minutes and we can consider one of the great dream mysteries (amnesia) to be tentatively solved: it is the joint product of the global aminergic demodulation that affects the entire brain and the more local disenablement of the dedicated circuitry of the dorsolateral prefrontal cortex that, in waking, allows us to be critical, decisive, and executive.

This is perhaps the most graphic example of how well the subtraction strategy of the mind-brain isomorphism strategy can work. Not only does it provide us with a plausible working hypothesis about the most conspicuous defects of dream consciousness, but it utilizes those defects to double back on and reinforce the positive contributions of the dorsolateral prefrontal cortex in waking. Furthermore, it prompts us to wonder if there may not be some unanticipated mechanistic link between the global neuromodulatory changes and the local cortical activation patterns that distinguish REM sleep from waking. What might that link be?

Cortico-Limbic Interactions

Long before PET scan studies revealed the dramatic shift in cortico-limbic balance (in favor of the limbic system in REM), affective neuroscientists like Richard Davidson had proposed just such shifts to account for data describing differences in the experience and expression of positive and negative affects. Some people are optimistic and outgoing, whereas others are pessimistic and introverted. Davidson's work has begun to explain these differences in terms of differential brain activation.

The Davidson hypothesis is complex because it has not just two but four components: the left vs. the right and top (cortex) vs. the bottom (limbic areas). Oversimplifying for the sake of clarity, preferential activation of the left prefrontal area is associated with positive dispositional affects like affections and optimism, whereas preferential activation of the right prefrontal area is associated with negative dispositional affects like social fearfulness and pessimism.

Because the affects themselves—especially fear—involve the limbic amygdala, it has been proposed that the left prefrontal cortex is more effective than the right in inhibiting the limbic sources of negative affect.

Imaging studies of regional brain activation within and across subjects during waking have confirmed this hypothesis.

We do not yet know if the left-right differences in cortical activation (measured in the waking EEG by Davidson) will persist, or be nullified, or even reversed in REM sleep, but we do know that compared to waking, the amygdala and its directly adjacent cortical areas, the parahippocampal and anterior cingulate regions, are selectively activated in REM sleep and, as discussed in the previous section, that this preferential limbic activation is reciprocal to deactivation of both dorsolateral prefrontal cortices.

This shift in regional brain activation maps onto the shift in the conscious experience of increased, often unbearably intense negative affect in REM sleep dreams. As I have related earlier, a study of dream emotion in normal subjects revealed that dreaming is associated with high levels of anxiety and anger. These two high survival but unpalatable emotions far outweigh the more pleasurable elation that is sometimes present. It is this data that leads me to suggest that most dreams are "bad trips" in the language of the psychedelic elation seekers. It may just be that the dreaming brain is tilted in the direction of negative affect and that drugs that tilt the brain in the direction of REM will therefore be more likely to trigger negative emotions like fear and anger than more highly valued positive emotions like elation, joy, affection, and eros.

How and why is the limbic forebrain selectively activated in REM so as to produce this kind of affective experience? The how answer is that in addition to its major cholinergic innervation from the basal forebrain the limbic area receives a direct projection from the dorsolateral pontine tegmentum, where the cholinergic neurons that become selectively active in REM sleep are found in animals. PET studies can't yet tell us if this particular brain stem region is selectively activated in human REM sleep, but we hypothesize that such a homology is likely.

The answer to the why question is more speculative, but it unites three important ideas. One idea is that negative affect is conservative, in that it is linked to threat (anxiety, anger) and loss (sadness). A second possibility is that depression may comprise all three negative affects. And a third idea is that depression and its negative affects are cholinergically enhanced (and aminergically suppressed). In this view, REM sleep maintains, and in so doing stimulates, our most extreme emotional defense systems so that we are constantly prepared for the worst possible fates.

The hypothesis of selective amygdala activation in REM could help account for the limbic domination of the cortex and the negative affect domination of dream consciousness simply by strengthening the temporal lobe structures in a relative sense. This might, in and of itself, result in dorsolateral prefrontal cortex deactivation via reciprocal inhibition. But it also seems possible—and even probable—that the shift in brain stem modulation from aminergic (in waking) to cholinergic (in REM) could also directly affect regional cortical activation and blood flow.

The truth of the matter is that we do not know how local cerebral blood flow is controlled so as to deliver oxygen to neuronal groups according to their needs. When, for example, I shift my attention from the stimuli in my environment to concentrated thought, how is the necessary redistribution of blood flow (from the back of my brain to the front) effected? And when I switch from waking to dreaming, how does the reverse change in blood flow (from front to back) occur? Some scientists think that all of the control is local, but it seems likely that at least some control would be central. The great advantage of a central control mechanism is that both neuronal activity *and* blood flow could be coordinated by the same physiological process.

To substantiate this central control hypothesis, we would need to show that the distribution of cholinergic axonal terminals was significantly different from that of the two aminergic neuronal groups. The most obvious way in which this is true is that whereas the two aminergic groups project widely and directly to many parts of the forebrain, including the cortex, the two brain stem cholinergic neuronal groups project directly only to the subcortical forebrain.

All of the cholinergic projection neurons that reach the cerebral cortex lie in the basal forebrain, and they too are without doubt secondarily activated during REM. I say "without doubt" because acetylcholine release from the cortex generally is as high in REM sleep as it is in waking and the basal forebrain cholinergic neurons are its only possible source. But what about possible regional differentiation of release? Regional microdialysis studies of acetylcholine release in waking (when norepinephrine and serotonin are also released) and in REM (when they are not) are now needed to answer this question.

At stake here is not only the mechanistic basis of differential selective brain activation patterns in different conscious states, but also the deeper question of how local neuronal activity and the cerebral microcirculation (1) are co-controlled, and (2) interact cooperatively. It would be surprising if the neuromodulators did not play an integrative role in this process.

The Direction of Consciousness and Content Selection

We are now in a position to speculate a bit more informedly about two related and age-old questions that have vexed psychology, philosophy, and religion since time immemorial. To what degree do we control the direction (or flow) of consciousness, and to what degree do we select its content? Put another way, to what extent are we rational creatures obeying an eighteenth-century enlightenment model and to what extent are we more instinctual automatons fulfilling a nineteenth-century anarchic model? These two models are conjoined in Freud's psychoanalytic model, which clearly favored the instinctual unconscious but expressed it in highly rationalistic terms. Are we now in a stronger position to advance this discussion?

If we point to the specifications of the brain basis of intellect vs. instinct, the answer is a resounding yes. We see, most clearly in the case of waking vs. dreaming consciousness, how the brain's overall chemical states and how its associated regional emphasis shift in ways that give us, for the first time in human history, a blueprint for the scientific psychology that Freud envisaged.

And the answer is "yes" if we emphasize the way the new findings enable us to revise Freud's necessarily speculative dream theory and replace it with one that gives a detailed alternative account of dream phenomenology and eliminates the very dubious disguise-censorship idea, but still retains the crucial concept of emotional salience as a major element in dream content elaboration. The model does not now specify regional shifts in neuronal activity and/or blood flow, but if both derive from the neuromodulatory ratio shift, then factor M would predict the enhancement of emotion in dreaming and its central role in shaping dream plots.

And the answer is "yes" if we enunciate the attendant notion of instinct and emotion as critically integral and adaptive to survival and reproduction rather than regarding them as anarchic and regressive. The difficult trick here is to achieve a balanced model of conscious and unconscious forces that will enable us to construct a new view of ourselves as possessing *both* the capacity to react rapidly and uncritically to stimuli and to reflect slowly and critically on our situation in the world.

As for the details needed to flesh out a new model, we must admit that there is more of an opportunity within our reach than there is substantial information in hand. The time is thus ripe for a major program of research that uses our now extensive knowledge of how conscious and unconscious processes are naturally generated and regulated in the diurnal evolution of our states of brain and mind as a foundation for a new comprehensive theory that encompasses the comparative, the evolutionary developmental, intra- and interindividual, and the social levels of analysis.

7

Models of Conscious State Alteration

The ability to map, even tentatively, from the level of cells and molecules up through the level of brain regions to the level of conscious experience depends upon having valid animal surrogates for the phenomena of interest. For most of the phenomena of interest the criterion cannot be met: we do not know if subhuman mammals suffer from states akin to schizophrenia, and we don't even know if they become "demented" as they age. But we do know that they possess such rudiments of consciousness as sensation, perception, emotion, and learning, and it is clear that all of these components of consciousness change state as these mammals go to sleep. In fact, the outward behavioral and deeper physiological manifestations of waking and sleep are so strikingly homologous as to suggest identity at the level of fundamental mechanisms.

It is the goal of this chapter to review what we know about those homologies, with a view to elaborating general models of conscious state change that lend themselves to the explanation of spontaneous changes in consciousness—like those that distinguish dreaming from waking and those that "alter" waking, especially by the introduction of drugs that interact with the neurons that regulate consciousness via natural chemicals and the cell membrane receptors with which they have affinity.

The Mammalian Sleep-Wake Cycle

The capacity to thermoregulate—to maintain body temperature within very narrow limits—is one of the great fundamental achievements of class mammalia. A complex variety of brain mechanisms guarantees this stability, and the brain, in turn, appears to be the principal beneficiary of thermal homeostasis. The experiences of febrile delirium and hypothermic disorientation—both of which have affected anyone who has ever spiked a fever of 105 degrees when battling the flu or suffered bad weather above the tree line in the mountains—tells us that those brain circuits upon which our coveted conscious experience depends are markedly thermolabile.

Thermoregulation and sleep are mutually enhancing, and we need to know much more about how and why. How, for example, is thermoregulation abandoned in REM sleep—the most essentially mammalian state of them all—and what purpose is served by allowing—and even forcing—the brain into a state akin to delirium and dementia? It is irresistible to assume that such high-risk tampering with thermal and cerebral homeostasis must have some very valuable payoff for consciousness. Maintaining the delicate balance of neural networks is one possibility; jostling the information in them in the interest of more efficient and salient filing is another. These are the great unanswered questions of sleep research today. But short of answering them precisely, we have learned a lot about how consciousness is altered in a thermally responsible way. The fact that all mammals have REM sleep means not only that they all share the mechanisms and benefits of that state, but also that any one species is an experimental model for the others. For a wide variety of reasons, the experimental models for sleep research have been cats (for cellular studies) and rats (for behavioral and pharmacological studies).

Circadian Rest-Activity Cycle

Our ups and our downs of behavioral output ride a wave of internal body temperature that mirrors the diurnal fluctuations of temperature that follow the sun's rising and setting. Light, of course, is symphonically orchestrated in the cosmic world of day and night and tells us even consciously what thermal time it is more clearly and crisply than hot/cold sensitivity.

In anticipatory response to these vital signals denoting energy and information availability to mammals, the brain has designed a clock for itself. Tinkered up from the biochemical rhythmicity of metabolic processes that change direction as temperature rises and falls, the mammalian circadian clock has come to be independent of temperature and it has been sequestered in two small nuclei sitting in the hypothalamus just above the optic chiasm. Unbeknownst to us, this clock controls the ebb and flow of our body temperature and energy, and with them, our tendency to be in a waking, sleeping, or dreaming state of consciousness.

When the circadian clock says "Act Now," it initiates a process that includes the activation of neuromodulatory cells in the brain stem. These cells, strategically located in the noradrenergic locus coeruleus and the serotonergic raphé, constitute what Vernon Mountcastle called "a brain within the brain," because their activity (in waking) or inactivity (in REM sleep) make such a difference to the brain's mode of operation. So important are they that they must be accorded a key role in any model that attempts to account for spontaneous and drug-induced alterations in consciousness.

Later in this chapter I will assign to them (and their cholinergic colleagues in the laterodorsal tegmental and pedunculopontine nuclei) one of three dimensions in the AIM state space model that I use to integrate the pharmacologically altered states with those that occur naturally. It is of paramount importance to emphasize that the brain uses its own chemical systems to achieve a rich panoply of altered states of consciousness, including some truly psychedelic ones!

The mechanism by which the circadian clock in the hypothalamus regulates the monoaminergic cells of the brain stem is poorly understood, but it appears to involve a direct inhibitory pathway that shuts down the locus coeruleus and raphé nuclei as part of a more complicated and guided set of "Don't Act Now" instructions. Interestingly, this inhibitory process is normally switched on only gradually, resulting in the orderly progression of states from drowsiness, through frank sleepiness, sleep onset, and then remarkable downward slide into deep NREM sleep.

This downward slide, which parallels the progressive throttling of the monoaminergic neurons by descending GABAergic inhibition, is accompanied by massive and global deactivation of the brain and body. As muscle tone declines, movement of all kinds becomes increasingly unlikely and, simultaneously, the threshold of response to external sensory stimulation rises. As cerebral tone declines, the thalamocortical system moves from its high frequency (desynchronized) to its low frequency (synchronized) mode of operation. As it does so, the electroencephalogram shows shifts through a spectrum of patterns reflecting the burst-pause firing of thalamocortical nerves, first as EEG spindles and later as high-voltage slow waves that bring the brain as close to oblivion as it ever normally gets. Naturally, mental activity also plummets dramatically.

So far, a unidimensional activation-deactivation model will suffice. Turn off the circadian clock and down goes everything. This is the turning off of the lights in the brain that Sherrington celebrated with his loom-shuttle metaphor of sleep and that can now be seen directly as the global decline in blood flow that PET images appropriately represent as dark blue and green, in contrast to the reds, yellows, and oranges that represent activation.

And, until recently, unidimensional activation models were widely promulgated as the linear sleep graphs that became the universal idioms of natural conscious state alterations. According to those graphs, the subsequent and periodically recurrent reversals of this downward trend that resulted in REM sleep could be understood and represented as reactivations of the brain. And this is true, but only in an electrical sense. As measured by the EEG, the brain *is* reactivated; the spindles and slow waves are suppressed and replaced by low voltage fast activity, including the gamma frequency 30–80 cycles per second pattern that has been touted as denoting sufficient temporal coherence among the widespread neuronal circuits of the cortex to permit the binding necessary for the unification of conscious experience.

But the activation-only model and the unidimensional graphs are inadequate because they do not represent either the active suppression of sensory input and motor output that is essential to the maintenance of behavioral sleep in the face of the restituted electrical activation state of the brain or the complete suppression of firing by locus coeruleus and raphe neurons that causes the electrically reactivated to become aminergically demodulated.

With these two important modifications, the brain has been put off line (by the gating of input and output) and had its mode of processing changed (by the modulatory shift), and is thus *de*activated both informationally and dispositionally. Models that fail to appreciate these important departures are doomed to factual error and lead to an interpretive narrowness that cannot begin to deal with the differentiations of conscious experience that are part and parcel of the processes under discussion.

To accommodate the effects on the activated brain of pulling it off-line with respect to its external inputs and outputs, and to recognize the fact that this gating does not parallel the electrical activation of the brain in REM, I have assigned the second dimension of the three dimensional AIM model, the dimension I, to input-output gating. In the case of factor I, we have an elaborately detailed picture of the cellular and molecular mechanisms that are called into play during REM sleep.

The sensory isolation of the brain is achieved via presynaptic inhibition of the Ia afferent terminals, the endings of the sensory nerves that form synapses with neurons in the brain itself. This process thus blocks the signals carrying representations of the external world into the brain. It appears to come from the same brain stem source, the pontomedullary reticular formation, that hyperpolarizes the motoneurons, rendering them less responsive to internally generated motor commands. The neuronal circuits mediating these and other changes during REM are schematically represented in figure 7.1.

The net result is that in one brain-activated state, waking, the brain is in touch with the outside world and can act upon it, whereas in another equally activated state, REM sleep, it cannot do either. In both cases, the activation is real and important and must constitute a dimension of any model. But so diametrically opposed are the input-output conditions of waking and REM that they cannot possibly be dealt with by an activation-only model. We need the input-output (I-O) dimension.

But even this necessary modification does not go far enough, because it does not (yet) specify where the information that *is* processed by the off-line, activated brain comes from or how that processing is actually organized. Two questions arise: (1) Does the activated brain simply churn out internal elements willy-nilly and process them as if they came from the outside world? Or (2), is there a more specific mechanism of internal input generation and a more specific mechanism of processing that gives the brain some advantage in its task of adaptation to the world? The answer to both questions is yes. The brain *is* specialized such that REM sleep is markedly different from waking in both its information generating and its information processing mechanisms. We now take each of these issues up in turn.

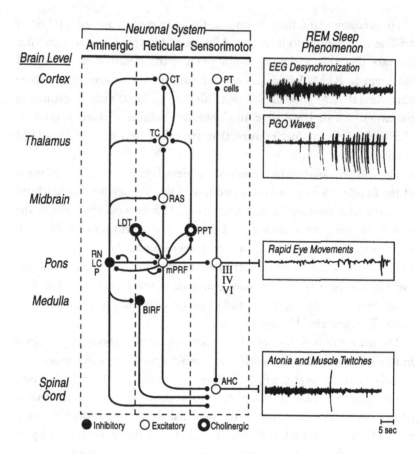

Figure 7.1
Schematic representation of the REM sleep generation process. A distributed network involves cells at many brain levels (left). The network is represented as comprising three neuronal systems (center) that mediate REM sleep electrographic phenomena (right). Postulated inhibitory connections are shown as solid circles; postulated excitatory connections as open circles; and cholinergic pontine nuclei are shown as open circles with darkened boundaries. It should be noted that the actual synaptic signs of many of the aminergic and reticular pathways remain to be demonstrated, and, in many cases, the neuronal architecture is known to be far more complex than indicated here (e.g., the thalamus and cortex). During REM, additive facilitatory effects on pontine REM-on cells are postulated to occur via disinhibition (resulting from the marked reduction in firing rate by aminergic neurons at REM sleep onset) and through excitation (resulting from mutually excitatory cholinergic-noncholinergic cell interactions within the pontine tegmentum). The net result is strong tonic and phasic activation of reticular and sensorimotor neurons in REM sleep. REM sleep phenomena are postulated to be mediated as follows: EEG desynchronization results from a net tonic increase

An Internal Pulse Generator for the Brain in REM Sleep: The PGO System

Studies with cats show that the very earliest sign of an oncoming REM period is the elaboration of very large spike and wave potentials in the EEG, recorded from the lateral geniculate bodies of the thalamus. These waves correspond to depolarization of the geniculate neurons by excitatory impulses arising not in the retina (as would be the case for waking visions), but in the pontine brain stem, where they also correspond to depolarization arising, apparently spontaneously, in neurons of the reticular formation and the pedunculopontine (PPT) region. Because the latter neurons fire in intense clusters *before* the waves are recorded, the PPT is thought to be the point of origin of these entirely endogenous signals. Because the signals originate in the pons (P) and radiate rostrally to the geniculate bodies (G) and also to the occipital cortex (O), they were called PGO waves by Jouvet, who first appreciated their significance.

Let me emphasize that these findings clearly demonstrate that the brain can generate its own information, independent of any external inputs, simply by changing the excitability of certain of its component neurons. In this case, the pontine neurons that become hyperexcitable almost certainly include the cholinergic elements of the PPT, and there is abundant evidence indicating that the PGO waves can be experimentally induced

in reticular, thalamocortical, and cortical neuronal firing rates. PGO waves are the result of tonic disinhibition and phasic excitation of burst cells in the lateral pontomesencephalic tegmentum. Rapid eye movements are the consequence of phasic firing by reticular and vestibular cells; the latter (not shown) directly excite oculomotor neurons. Muscular atonia is the consequence of tonic postsynaptic inhibition of spinal anterior horn cells by the pontomedullary reticular formation. Muscle twitches occur when excitation by reticular and pyramidal tract motorneurons phasically overcomes the tonic inhibition of the anterior horn cells. Abbreviations: RN, raphé nuclei; LC, locus coeruleus; P, peribrachial region; PPT, pedunculopontine tegmental nucleus; LDT, laterodorsal tegmental nucleus; mPRF, meso- and mediopontine tegmentum (e.g., gigantocellular tegmental field, parvocellular tegmental field); RAS, midbrain reticular activating system; BIRF, bulbospinal inhibitory reticular formation (e.g., gigantocellular tegmental field, parvocellular tegmental field, magnocellular tegmental field); TC, thalamocortical; CT, cortical; PT cell, pyramidal cell; III, oculomotor; IV, trochlear; V, trigminal motor nuclei; AHC, anterior horn cell. (From Hobson et al., 2000, *Behavioral and Brain Sciences* 23) by local cholinergic microstimulation. This means that the chemical nature of this internal signal system is both known and controllable, a huge advance with numerous scientific implications.

We can also specify the mechanism by which the pontine PGO generator becomes cholinergically hyperexcitable: it is the withdrawal of serotonergic inhibition and neuromodulation that results from shutting down the raphé nucleus serotonin containing neurons that itself results from the "Don't Act Now" signals sent down into the pons from the hypothalamic circadian clock. The net result of the cholinergic hyperexcitability is, however, to alter the brain—and with it consciousness—so that instead of really acting, it only imagines it is doing so. We need to look more closely at this concept, which has a strong bearing on the way that psychoactive drugs affect our brains and our conscious experience.

"Fictive movement" is movement that is centrally commanded but peripherally inhibited. We already know about the peripheral inhibition: it is the hyperpolarization of the final common path motoneurons by "no go" signals from the brain stem. The movement commands arise at many levels of the pyramidal and extrapyramidal motor system, including the motor pattern generator circuits of the pons itself (which can initiate stepping and other gaits with or without being told to do so by the higher centers) and by cortical pyramidal tract neurons (which fire in intense clusters during REM just as they do when they command movement in waking). Other motor structures that may be involved in creating the almost perfect illusion of movement that fills all of our REM sleep dreams are the pontine gray, the cerebellum, the red nucleus, the basal ganglia, and our old friend the thalamus.

That adverse consequences would arise—were it not for the active inhibition of movement—is made dramatically clear by patients who lose their innate ability to block other motor outputs and hence enact their sometimes self-injurious dream scenarios. We will come back to this story when we discuss the tendency of some legally prescribed, consciousness altering drugs to mimic those CNS degenerative diseases that cause this so-called REM sleep behavior disorder. The one motor system whose REM sleep activation results in real, not fictive movement is, of course, the one that moves the eyes rapidly, giving REM its name. There is no need to inhibit *this* system, because its motor output creates no behavioral disruption of sleep or other adverse consequences for the dreamer.

A possible link between the movement of the eyes (which is real) and the hallucinated dream movements (which are fictive) is provided by the PGO system. This is because the neuronal firing patterns associated with each PGO wave encode (at least) the direction of the eye movements and provide that encoded information to (at least) the visual thalamus and visual cortex. This means that in the absence of real sensory input from the eyes, feed forward information about the direction of the (also fictive) gaze is provided to the upper brain, which could (and we think almost certainly must) use it in the elaboration of the convincing visuomotor illusion that is dreaming.

There are two reasons for taking this idea seriously. One is that the vestibulo-cerebellar system, which is intimately involved in tracking and coordinating the movement of our body in space, is an integral part of the PGO system. The other is that in waking, PGO-like activity is generated in reaction to novel stimuli that provoke the startle response, a highly coordinated and complex set of head, neck, trunk, and limb movements that serve to orient us to the stimulus needing our evaluation and action. In both examples we see that the PGO waves may be more than a mere copy of eye movement—they may be a command signal for a whole set of organized visuomotor behaviors.

It has been proposed—I think not entirely facetiously—that dreaming is our subjective awareness of an uninterrupted sequence of startle responses. There are two attractive aspects of this hypothesis: the first is that it is congruous with our emotional experience of dreams, that strange combination of wonder and surprise with anxiety and fear, as if we were constantly being jolted by stimuli that were they to occur in response to real world signals on waking would provoke shock and even panic. This idea has its own internal support in the finding that PGO signals travel to the emotion processors in the amygdala, as well as to the visuomotor brain.

The second is that the startle hypothesis could also link sensorimotor orientation to cognitive orientation, and by constantly forcing a resetting of the former system wreak havoc with the latter. This would help us understand the orientational instability at the root of dream bizarreness. By orientational instability, I mean the tendency for dream people, places, times, and actions to be discontinuous and/or incongruous, as if the brain-mind system could never settle on a stable, internally consistent set of albeit fictive parameters. It is precisely this quality of dreams that many modern artists have used to create troubling images (like René Magritte's paintings and the scenarios of Alain Renais's films).

I believe that the cognitive uncertainty of dreams has still deeper roots that lie in the problem that REM sleep brain chemistry poses for memory construction, but the fact remains that REM sleep consciousness depends upon and must take account of sequences of internal signals that, by their very nature, cannot be expected to have continuity and congruity because they constantly tell the brain "Hey, watch out, something new and unexpected is going on!" And the poor mind struggling to fit the new data with the old sometimes achieves remarkable coherence under these very adverse working conditions. We will see that drugs that drive the system in the direction of REM sleep create similar difficulties for cognitive integration.

The Heart of the Brain: Neuromodulation and Aminergic-Cholinergic Interaction

Long before the circadian system and its influence on the sleep cycle was appreciated, Walter Hess had proposed the concept of a balanced alternation between active and restorative physiological states based upon sympathetic-parasympathetic reciprocity. Hess had won a Nobel Prize for his work in the 1930s and 1940s on the effects of brain stimulation on behavior and autonomic nervous system physiology. He conceived of an ergotrophic mode, mediated by the sympathetic side of his model, which favored the waking state and all of those energy-consuming behavioral acts that occur within it; and a trophotropic mode, mediated by the cholinergic side of his model, which favored sleep and all of those energy restorative functions that it favors.

Hess's model is all the more prescient because, at the time of its articulation, the cellular and molecular neurobiology of the central instantiation of the two branches of the autonomic nervous system were completely unknown. He had to infer their existence from his knowledge of the peripheral system and from the effects of his manipulation of the brain upon their outflow. The breakthrough came only in the early 1960s, when Anica Dahlstrom, Kjell Fuxe, and others identified the norepinephrine containing cells of the locus coeruleus and the serotonin containing cells of the midline raphé nucleus. And it was even later when Marcel Mesulam and others mapped the central cholinergic neuronal system.

By 1970, it was clear that the brain contained a wide variety of chemically specific neuronal subtypes that were capable not only of a diverse panoply of short-term effects on other neurons, but also of possibly exerting such effects over the much longer time scale of enduring states like waking and sleep. This concept—of neuromodulation as a special form of neurotransmission—took root when it was tied to the second messenger idea, and is still evolving as even a third messenger system is being discovered. The term "messenger" denotes the molecules involved in a chain of signals, as follows: (1) neurotransmission and neuromodulation (first messengers); (2) translation of the above messages into intracellular commands (second messengers); and (3) translation of above signals into metabolic gene products such as enzymes (third messengers).

Because the neuromodulators trigger metabolic events that extend beyond the membrane (via second messengers) to the genetic machinery of the nucleus (generating third messengers), their spontaneous fluctuations over the sleep-wake cycle and their manipulation by psychoactive drugs creates effects that in space and time can become the substrates of adaptive (and maladaptive) functions that are both global and enduring. They can, for example, help us understand how and why sleep affects mood and why drugs that alter sleep also alter mood and vice versa. Similarly, they can help us understand the long-term effects of sleep on cognitive function and how and why drugs that affect sleep may benefit or impair cognitive capacities.

Reciprocal Interaction Between Cholinergic REM-On and Aminergic REM-Off Cells

Because it was known by 1960 that the pontine brain stem was crucial to REM sleep generation, it was natural to assume that the newly discovered modulatory elements played an important role in its generation. It was even reasonable, on an *a priori* basis, that each of the elements had responsibility for one state, *viz*, dopamine controls waking, serotonin controls slow wave sleep, and norepinephrine controls REM. Early lesion and parenteral pharmacological studies—some even armed with measures of amine concentrations in the brain—gave initial support to this concept. For example, Michel Jouvet produced insomnia in cats by blocking the enzyme that is essential to convert tryptophane into serotonin. He interpreted this result to mean that serotonin was a sleep mediator.

But single-cell recording and local microinjection studies soon showed that the three pontine neuromodulators interact in a far more complex and versatile fashion. In waking, all of them can be activated; in NREM sleep, all of them tend to be deactivated; in REM sleep, the two aminergic systems are completely deactivated, with the cholinergic system hyperactivated. This unexpected result shows that although REM sleep is wake-like in its EEG aspect, it is not only off line informationally speaking, but probably also processing its information differently by virtue of the radical shift to exclusive cholinergic modulation. This proposition also suggests that because it is so predominantly cholinergic, REM sleep, which Walter Hess didn't know existed, may be much more trophotropic than many of its superficial physiological signs would suggest. To illustrate this point, I consider it paradoxical—and counterintuitive—to suggest that the strong central (EEG) and peripheral (blood pressure, respiration, and heart rate) activation processes favor rest and restoration. Just the opposite would appear to be the case because, in waking, these same signs are associated with stress and the famous fight or flight response. The paradox is resolved, however, if we realize that although we might dream of fleeing or fighting, we don't actually fight or fly, so the energy expenditure is minimal. Meanwhile, cells in the depths of the brain *are* resting and restoring themselves for the ergotropic tasks of tomorrow.

We can readily appreciate that because the neuromodulatory systems diverge in such radical ways between waking and sleep, they do not obey the simple activation rule any more than input-output gating functions do. They must therefore be accorded a special functional place in models of conscious state alteration.

That is why the AIM model assigns one of its three dimensions, M, to modulation. For the sake of simplicity, it expresses the ratio of cholinergic to aminergic neuromodulator release. Before going into a detailed description of the AIM model, I should point out that although the activation is clearly discordant with both input-output gating and with modulation, the latter two functions track one another quite well. When the system is most strongly exteroceptive in waking it is strongly aminergic, and when it is most powerfully interoceptive (in REM sleep) it is strongly cholinergic. This reciprocal interaction between the aminergic and cholinergic systems is shown in figure 7.2.

The mapping of function I onto function M suggests some as yet poorly understood link between sensorimotor orientation and chemical predisposition. What could that link possibly be? The first answer that comes to mind is that the PGO system is, as we have seen, intrinsically cholinergic. That is to say, the internal pulse generator is a cholinergic pulse generator that contains not only spatiotemporal codes, but also processing instructions for them. Because of the identity of the PGO system with the startle network, it seems possible that what the pulse generator is saying is, "save this information because it is important." In other words, the system uses some of the same rules to establish processing priorities in both waking (when real life events are being processed on-line) and in dreaming (when some of them are being reprocessed off-line).

Experimental Evidence

The crucial experiments suggesting these novel concepts were begun in the late 1960s, became fully developed in the mid-1970s, and continue to be fruitful today.

The extracellular microelectrode recording technique developed by David Hubel for his epochal studies of the cat visual system and further perfected by Eduard Evarts for his pioneering work on the cat motor system was easily applied to exploring the brain stem. There were two major obstacles that needed to be overcome to guarantee success, however. The first was movement: not only was head movement itself a problem, but body movement also had to be limited because the targets were deep and located on the major axis of lateral and vertical head-on-neck movement. The second problem was identification of the neurons of interest. At the onset, no one knew that the modulatory elements would identify themselves both by their distinctive spike-to-spike firing pattern, but also—and this is the main point of the discovery—by their dramatic state dependent alterations of firing propensity.

The interesting neurons were small and few, but there were enough of them that were big enough to make themselves known even to experimenters like us, who had no idea what to expect from them! Call it persistence, or call it luck that we found them, but certainly call it opportunism that we knew what to do with them. Perhaps the most important lesson in this story is that the brain, for all of its complexity, is also simple. One

A. Structural Model

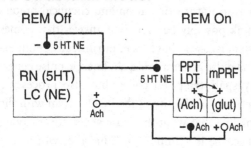

B. Dynamic Model

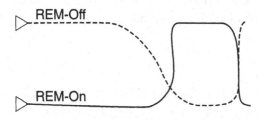

C. Activation Level (A)

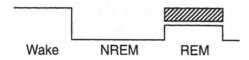

Figure 7.2
The Reciprocal Interaction Model of physiological mechanisms determining alterations in activation level. (A) Structural model of reciprocal interaction with synaptic modifications of the original model based on recent findings. As in the original model, pontine REM-off cells are noradrenergically (NE) or serotonergically (5HT) inhibitory (−) at their synapses. In the original model, REM-on cells of the pontine reticular formation were cholinoceptively excited and/or cholinergically excitatory at their synaptic endings, while the model shown here depicts recently reported self-inhibitory (−) cholinergic (Ach) autoreceptors in mesopontine cholinergic nuclei and the mutually excitatory (+) interactions between mesopontine cholinergic and noncholinergic (glut) neurons. Note that the exponential magnification of cholinergic output predicted by the original model can also occur in the model depicted here with mutually excitatory cholinergic-noncholinergic interactions taking the place of the previously postulated, mutually excitatory cholinergic-cholinergic interactions. In the revised model, inhibitory cholinergic autoreceptors would contribute to the inhibition of LDT and PPT cholinergic neurons, which is also caused by noradrenergic and serotonergic inputs to these nuclei. Therefore the originally proposed shape of reciprocal interaction's dy-

should be able to guess this: if the brain wants to instantiate a set of highly reliable, stereotyped, and automatic operating conditions—like REM sleep, for example—it is going to utilize a mechanism that is reliable, stereotyped, and automatic to achieve it. Even if you don't know exactly what you are looking for, keep poking around, and sooner or later, you will stumble on a secret!

To us, it happened twice: once when we unwittingly probed the locus coeruleus looking for REM-on cells and found, by mistake, our first REM-off cells; and later, when we were looking for more REM-off cells in the peribrachial region of the lateral pons, and discovered instead the most impressive REM-on cells we had ever seen, the PGO burst cells.

The first observation was the more unexpected because we were under the mistaken impression that the locus coeruleus should turn on, not off, in REM. But once we realized that we had the role of norepinephrine backwards, it was not difficult to find other REM-off cells—not only in the locus coeruleus, but also in the raphé nuclei—and to see that both of the pontine aminergic neuromodulators supported waking just as any extension of Hess's principles would suggest. Even the central sympathetic system works toward ergotrophic ends. For sleep to occur, this system must first be deactivated to allow NREM sleep to develop, and then actively suppressed, to allow REM to develop.

We were primed to make the second observation because we knew that the peribrachial region was sensitive to cholinergic microstimulation and that it contained the cellular progenitors of the PGO waves that were

namic model and its resultant alternation of behavioral state also result from this revised model. (B) Dynamic model. During waking the pontine aminergic (dashed line) system is tonically activated and inhibits the pontine cholinergic (solid line) system. During NREM sleep aminergic inhibition gradually wanes and cholinergic excitation reciprocally waxes. At REM sleep onset aminergic inhibition is shut off and cholinergic excitation reaches its high point. (C) Activation level. As a consequence of the interplay of the neuronal systems shown in (A) and (B), the net activation level of the brain (A) is at equally high levels in waking and REM sleep and at about half this peak level in NREM sleep. Abbreviations: open circles, excitatory influences; filled circles, inhibitory influences; RN, dorsal raphé nucleus; LC, locus coeruleus; mPRF, medial pontine reticular formation; PPT, pedunculopontine tegmental nucleus; LDT, laterodorsal tegmental nucleus; 5HT, serotonin; NE, norepinephrine; Ach, acetylcholine; glut, glutamate. (From Hobson et al., 2000, *The New Cognitive Neurosciences*, M. Gazzaniga ed., MIT Press) produced, by the millions, when we put carbachol into that area. The peribrachial region contains the peduculopontine nucleus that produces acetylcholine, which we think may mediate the PGO waves. Carbachol is a synthetic molecule that looks like acetylcholine to the cells it contacts but—because it is not acetylcholine—it resists enzymatic breakdown and thus produces prolonged, intense enhancement of acetylcholine-like action. So when we recorded cells there that fired in clusters on the leading edge of each PGO wave, we knew we had found what we were looking for. But we did not anticipate that these cells would encode eye movement direction and forward that information to the lateral geniculate body (LGB), because no one had previously recognized the markedly lateralized aspect of LGB-PGO amplitudes!

This discovery was almost too good to be true. It meant that each PGO wave could serve not only as a timing pulse, but also as a unit of spatial information. Now we don't really know if PGO waves do either of these two important tasks, but synchronization of the brain by a pulse generator has to occur, as does the creation of internal models of the world. Before accepting these hypotheses as principles, we need to know whether humans also have a PGO system and what happens when that system is dissociated from the rest of the brain or disenabled.

Both dissociation and disenablement can already be achieved in animals. With respect to dissociation, the PGO waves that are evoked by cholinergic microstimulation with carbachol can be state independent in two experimental paradigms: short-term and long-term REM enhancement. By short term I mean four to six hours and by long term I mean six to ten days of altered function. The differences between the two syndromes appear to derive only from the very small distance between the two lateral brain stem sites from which they are evoked.

To produce short-term REM enhancement, we place the carbachol in many different areas of the pontine reticular formation. To produce long-term PGO enhancement, we place it farther back and more laterally (very near the anterior border of vestibular nuclei). The two syndromes are both unexpected and baffling, raising far more questions than they answer. In fact, the only clear answer that they give is that the lateral pons is a chemically specialized area whose activation can unleash enduring changes in brain function. We can therefore use this discovery as a possible bridge to understanding the equally surprising and baffling long-term nature of many psychoactive drug effects (and side effects). For example, we need a way of thinking about the emergence of the REM sleep behavior disorder during the long-term use of selective serotonin reuptake blockers (SSRIs) like fluoxetine (Prozac) and, even more important, why this unwanted pathology may persist long after discontinuance of the drug!

So we need to add the word "troubling" to the adjectives "surprising" and "baffling" when we talk about long-term drug effects. Most scientists who use a drug experimentally, most physicians who prescribe a drug chemically, and most laypersons who take a drug recreationally assume that the effects will be short-lived. They may be sadly mistaken. Indeed, we already talk about long-term drug users whose brains are fried, burnt out, or cooked. For example, persistent memory defects and sleep alterations have been reported following the use of MDMA (or "Ecstasy"), a neurotoxic serotonin releaser that is the current drug of choice among many young persons. But we also know that long-term use of legitimate drugs can cause alarming positive symptoms like the tardive dyskinesia that afflicts many schizophrenic patients after years of dopamine receptor blockade with antipsychotic medication.

As for disenabling the PGO system, the only means until now available is the destruction of neurons in the long-term enhancement zone. This approach is as unacceptable as it is infeasible. As a prospective treatment we do not yet contemplate introducing any drugs directly into the human brain, let alone cytotoxic ones. But these long-term experimental paradigms, discovered by chance, are strongly heuristic and encourage us to look more actively for other means of inducing them—and for other ways of thinking about them.

All of these inadvertent discoveries grew out of our experiments on short-term REM enhancement, a paradigm that matches perfectly the conventional models of drug time course that most of us use as scientists, physicians, and self-stimulators. When carbachol is placed in the pontine reticular formation, it causes a prompt (0.5–5 minutes) and brief (2–4 hours) increase in REM sleep. The increase is, however, as robust (100–400 percent) as it is in long-term REM enhancement, indicating that we are producing a major takeover of the state control systems of the brain. The target zone is much larger than the more lateral long-term REM enhancement sites, suggesting that the medial area is a trigger zone and the lateral area a control region. What neurobiological factors might underlie this difference?

The only answers that we can advance with confidence now are that the short-term syndrome probably reflects postsynaptic level effects. We use the term "downstream" to denote the remoteness in both space and time of the long-term effects and recognize that they will be much more difficult to track because we don't know exactly where to look for their mediating mechanisms. However, it seems probable that we will need molecular biological tools to identify these fascinating, powerful, and problematic processes.

During the LSD era, those scientists who worried about permanent consequences of habitual drug use were branded as alarmists. But we now see that even purportedly innocent drugs, whose clinical use is widely sanctioned, affect molecular-level events and influence the genes to increase or decrease their products for very long time spans. We need to know much more about the biochemistry of these cascades that turn milliseconds into hours, hours into days, and days into years.

A State-Space Model for Understanding How Consciousness Is Altered

Having sermonized so long and hard about the time dimension, I am embarrassed now to promote a model that practically ignores it! Time was the second dimension in activation-only models that plotted functions like EEG synchronization, desynchronization, muscle tone, eye movement, and autonomic measures as the first dimension. In the still traditional sleep charts, these functions rise and fall against time. In the three-dimensional model I will now develop, time is a fourth dimension, seen only as a sequence of points within the state space.

We can measure activation as a neural function (like reticular formation neuronal discharge or EEG frequency and amplitude), and for the purposes of this model we considered it to be global. Obviously this is an already outmoded assumption, because we know from PET that very significant differences in regional activities can occur with similar levels of global activation. But moving a three-dimensional model is as much as a visual analog can handle, and because we wonder if the regional differences may map onto one of the other dimensions, we put this issue on hold for the time being.

Whereas in the conventional 2-D schema, activation is displayed on the y-axis, in the 3-D schema it is displayed as the x-axis. Instead of going up and down, it goes from side to side. High activation states are thus on the right and low activation states on the left of the state space. By activation I mean to suggest the instantaneous energy level of the brain-mind system. When it is high, consciousness is vivid and intense. Information is rapidly processed. When it declines, as in NREM sleep, consciousness is dull and lethargic. Information processing is slow. When it nears zero, as in coma, consciousness is impossible. No information processing occurs. To visualize this model, see again figures 2.6, 2.7, and 2.8.

Conventional models only implied input-output gating. The models indicated eye movement as if it were constant in REM and didn't occur in waking. Muscle tone was sometimes used in scoring sleep records and its absence in diagnosing REM, but it was at least as often ignored, and exclusive reliance placed on EEG and eye movement criteria.

In the new model, we see input-output gating as the openness or porosity of the system to exchanges of information between the outside and inside. If the gates are open, as in waking, sensory stimuli have free access to the information-processing circuits of the brain and the motor commands that are issued or executed. When the gates are closed, external world stimuli are denied access and internally generated motor commands are blocked. The z-axis in the new model represents the condition of the I-O gates. Under this convention, we could say the I-O gating function goes forward (closed) or backward (open).

Another way of looking at this I-O function is as the balance of external and internal data that is processed. Obviously, thresholds to sensory input and motor output are always relative, never absolute (except in death). Even when the system is fully exteroceptive a great deal of internally generated data is processed; likewise, when the gates are maximally closed, some external information can enter the system and some motor commands can escape.

We can measure factor I as the threshold to arousal, as the amplitude of the spinal reflex or, because we want to know the intensity of internal stimulation, as the frequency of eye movement in the presence of complete somatomotor atonia. This measure is used as a proxy for putative PGO wave frequency. As such, it also constitutes an indirect estimate of cholinergic activity, which is, in turn, a measure of aminergic demodulation. This raises questions about the independence of Factor I and Factor M, the third dimension of the model. Neuromodulation (M) is the only dimension of the model that previous conceptualizations did not consider, even implicitly. This is because it cannot yet be measured in humans and is therefore entirely speculative with respect to human consciousness and to the modeling of its natural and artificial alterations. But we can be confident of the face validity of the dimension for two important reasons.

The first reason is homology. Because all mammals, including man, have homologous brain stems and homologous sleep cycles, it would be very surprising to find a functional dissociation across species of the aminergic decline and reciprocal cholinergic ascendance across the states of sleep.

The second reason is the coherence between the modulation (M) dimension of the model and the effects of drugs that affect the aminergic and cholinergic systems upon the sleep-wake cycle in humans. With a few important exceptions, it is generally true that aminergic agonists enhance waking at the expense of sleep, whereas aminergic antagonists promote sleep at the expense of waking. Because it has two major components, one in the brain stem and one in the basal forebrain, the cholinergic system is more complicated but, again, it is generally true that cholinergic agonists enhance REM and even dreaming in humans, whereas cholinergic antagonists block both.

Dimension M, the aminergic-cholinergic ratio, is the y-axis of the 3-D AIM model. As such, it takes the place of activation. This seems justified because M and only M can fully explain the physiological and psychological differences between the two brain-activated states of waking and dreaming. It is the most novel and important axis of the new conceptualization, and it will be the dimension that we will rely on most strongly as we discuss the abnormal and/or unwanted states that arise spontaneously in some humans and are affirmatively induced by drug taking in others.

At present, the aminergic drive (a) and cholinergic drive (c), giving the ratio $a/c = M$, can be directly measured only in animals, to date only in cats and rats. In these species individual neurons of the locus coeruleus, raphé nuclei, or pedunculopontine nucleus can be identified and recorded extracellularly as the behavioral states naturally evolve. These increases can be complimented by assays of norepinephrine, serotonin, and acetylcholine to show that the chemical assumptions based upon the cellular neurophysiology are valid. We must search rigorously for a proxy of M in man. Perhaps it will come via a combination of receptor labeling and imaging technology. Until then we must be content with informed speculation, because we cannot deal with the phenomenology without a chemical dimension like M.

8

Sleep and Dream Disorders

In order for dreaming to be contained in sleep, the brain must sharply demarcate its states. But it often fails to do so, as anyone who has awakened from a nightmare unable to move knows at first hand. The terror that prompted the awakening in the first place is not only unabated by the arousal, but it may be augmented as the return of waking consciousness takes account of the persistent sleep paralysis.

In fact, brain states are determined by so many interacting variables that it is remarkable there is as much coherence as we normally experience when passing from sleep to waking and from waking to sleep. The normality of dissociation of state components and the blurring of state boundaries are both easily understood and explained by the multidimensional AIM state space model.

In this chapter we will look at several examples of state boundary blurring and frank dissociations of state components with an eye to appreciating just how easy it is—even without drugs—to create unexpected hybrid states of consciousness. We will then be in a strong position to review and to more fully understand why drugs that alter neuromodulation—changing the M dimension of the state space—so frequently and so easily alter consciousness in the direction of dreaming.

Hypnogogic Hallucinations

One of the most instructive examples of state boundary crossing is the tendency to experience dreamlike visuomotor sensations at sleep onset. These are called hypnagogic hallucinations if the subject is still awake enough to notice or be aroused by them. Apparently, one need only carry waking brain activation over the sleep boundary and dreaming will im-

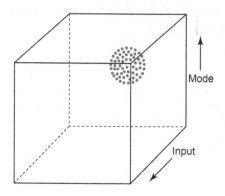

Figure 8.1
Hallucinations in waking (psychosis). When internal input strength exceeds that of external input, perceptual imagery is generated and integrated with the externally generated perceptions. The hallucinatory domain is on the right because activation remains high, and near the ceiling because aminergic drive is still strong (although some drugs may interfere with the naturally released neuromodulators).

mediately occur. In this case it seems very unlikely that the modulatory systems will have changed their absolute levels to those of REM sleep, but we do know from animal studies that attention lapses (or microsleeps, if you prefer) *are* associated with temporary cessations of aminergic neuronal firing. We will come back to this point later when we consider mediating mechanisms more carefully.

For any hallucination to arise, the perceptual system must become unbalanced in favor of internal stimuli. We already know from our consideration of the PGO system, that such shifts in balance are to be expected, given the fact that internal stimuli are constantly generated in the service of processing external ones. Thus there need only be a very slight decline in external input strength and/or a slight increase in internal stimulus strength to favor a takeover of the perceptual apparatus by internal stimuli. That making hallucinations is predominantly a function of changes in factor I is shown in figure 8.1.

This process is further favored by biasing the internal expectancy set as, for example, when the subject is not only sleepy but apprehensive. Conscious efforts to maintain vigilance, even under strenuous conditions, may be unavailing because of internal expectancy (let's call it priming) if the perceptual apparatus becomes both a motive force and a shaper of false perception.

To understand this mechanism directly, imagine yourself arriving home late at night to an empty house and finding the back door ajar. Your internal set is immediately on guard for an intruder and, as you enter the dark back hall, you can actually hear a muted thumping sound that you localize, roughly, to the front of the house on the second floor. Now the emotional arousal works to sharpen the focus of your attention. Your task is to explain the open door and the noise above. The obvious hypothesis is: intruder. It *pays* to expect the worst, and to learn, after an anxious five minutes, that the door was open because your housekeeper had neglected to close it securely when she left that morning and that the rustling sound was a loose shutter opened and closed by the light wind.

Meanwhile, your consciousness has run through an entire film archive of thriller fantasies. As in a dream, the diminished external cues, the heightened anxiety, and the reduced level of alertness conspire to call forth torrents of terror scenario. From jewel thief to serial killer, you check the file as you proceed from room to room and breathe a sigh of relief on finding each empty and undisturbed. "I was just imagining things," you say to yourself when you finally reach the bedroom and discover the errant shutter. Then you back-project to the open door and realize that today was Sonya's day to clean the house and that Sonya is such a fastidious housekeeper that she often forgets to put things back as she found them. And if that old door is not actively locked, it *can* blow open.

However relieved, and however exhausted, you are unlikely to be easily able to fall asleep without some resurgence of anxiety or altered perceptions. This is because falling asleep under any circumstance is characterized by the sudden eruption of dreamlike conscious experience. These sleep onset microdreams are often associated with classic jerks of the trunk and extremities akin to those in startle reactions. Reasoning teleologically, it would seem that nature had evolved a built-in burglar alarm system to provide us with a security check at sleep onset, just the time that we are about to become most vulnerable to predation!

In order for a sleep onset dream to become a hypnagogic hallucination, the internal stimulus strength has only to achieve a momentary advantage over the diminished force of external stimuli to generate emotionally salient perceptions. Because the prevalent emotion is anxiety, the salient imagery is fearsome, as befits the evolutionary theory advanced above. "Better safe than sorry," and "Forewarned is fore-armed," as we say.

This normalizing account of hypnagogic hallucinations lends itself nicely to explanation in terms of AIM and hence to integration with those spontaneous and induced alterations in conscious state that interest us most. For example, an exaggeration of the normal tendency to hallucinate at sleep onset is seen in narcolepsy, as well as with the use of clinical and recreational drugs that alter the M axis of the AIM model in ways that promote REM sleep phenomena, including the intense dreaming often associated with it.

Many narcoleptic patients show a marked intensification of sleep onset REM physiology, making the enhancement of hypnagogic hallucinations easily understandable. Because narcolepsy is also associated with the occurrence of hallucinations on awakening from REM sleep, I will defer discussion of the clinical aspects of the disorder until we have considered these hypnopompic extensions of dreaming into the wake state.

Hypnopompic Hallucinations

Whether we experience anxious dream perceptions on falling asleep or upon awakening, they are disturbing because they are quite correctly interpreted as psychotic processes. Everyone knows that psychosis is formally defined by the presence of hallucinations and delusions, and that psychosis is a sign of mental illness. What most people *don't* appreciate is that hypnagogic and hypnopompic hallucinations are *not* especially common in either schizophrenia or manic depressive mental illnesses, and that they denote a process whose physiology is so highly specific as to constitute an organic—that is to say neurological—basis of these symptoms.

But why are hypnopompic hallucinations even more unwelcome than hypnagogic ones? Probably because most people find that falling asleep is easily understood as a time of increasing disorder of the brain-mind and, as such, better tolerated because it is also a time of diminishing awareness of internal experience. Waking up, on the other hand, is a time when increasing orderliness is expected, and waking is followed by persistent awareness that allows critical self-reflection.

In the first case, the subject says, "Oh well, I was just falling asleep, so no wonder I had a vision; and then I became oblivious and couldn't worry about it anyway!" In the second case, the subject who wakes up hallucinating more properly associates the symptom with waking and says, "My God, I must be crazy if I am seeing things in my bedroom" (especially if it is in daylight).

I speak to this point from experience. Although I had little difficulty blowing off the imaginary intruder who used to come into my laboratory when I was about to doze off during all-night recordings, I could not so easily discount the man with the knife who stood over my bed when I woke up from my nightmare dream in Arizona.

Sleep, after all, is a state associated with dreaming, but waking is not. Even though the mechanism is likely the same in both cases, a failure to achieve a simultaneous and fully synchronous change in all of the components of consciousness that constitute states, we more easily accept sleep intrusions into waking at the exit portal.

Hypnopompic hallucinations clearly illustrate the continuation of REM sleep dreaming into subsequent waking. That is, instead of arising out of the blue (out of thin air, as we say), they simply continue an ongoing—and perfectly normal—sleep-related hallucinatory process across the line into waking. Practically everyone has had *some* experience with uncoordinated state transitions on arousal from sleep. Sleep walking, being unable to move, and persistent anxiety after arousal from a chase dream are some common examples.

But hypnopompic hallucinations may be more difficult to *accept* because their content is often more terrifying—or more bizarre—than those that accompany sleep onset. This is particularly true of those hypnopompic hallucinations associated with changing levels of neuromodulators when patients are trying to get off antidepressant and other psychoactive medications that powerfully interact with serotonergic and cholinergic brain mechanisms. The nightmares that some of these patients have are so terrifying that they do not even want to go to sleep because they so dread the awakenings.

One of my patients regularly had a ferocious alligator come out from under her bed and snap its teeth at her! This unwelcome bed partner *only* appeared when we were raising, or more commonly lowering, the patient's dose of amytriptyline, a tricyclic antidepressant that blocks the reuptake of the biogenic amines norepinephrine and serotonin (and so potentiates them) and also blocks the action of acetylcholine (and so enfeebles that system). Now that we know that REM sleep dreaming is driven by cholinergic neuromodulation and held in check by aminergic restraint, it seems unlikely that my patient's inability to contain her alligators within the confines of sleep—where they would more naturally have been forgotten—was related to the reciprocal effects of lowering the concentration of drug upon the two opposed intrinsic control systems. As the effects of amytriptyline wore off, the aminergic system weakened, decreasing the inhibitory restraint on the cholinergic system—which, because its pent-up energy was no longer countered, went into overdrive. We will return to this set of themes in chapter 11 when we discuss mood disorders and their treatment.

False Awakenings: Delusion on Top of Delusion

The interesting phenomenon of false awakening can also occur normally. Subjects who are expected to wake up promptly and unexpectedly from sleep are particularly prone to false awakening. In a false awakening, the subject dreams that he or she is awake, but is not. The delusion that one is awake, usually implicit in dreaming, now becomes explicit. Instead of simply assuming that I must be awake (because I am conscious, seeing and doing wake-like things), I now say, "Well I woke up the way I was supposed to do, fulfilled my obligation, and can now go back to sleep!"

I myself had this very disconcerting experience when I was an experimental subject in one of our early Nightcap studies conducted by Robert Stickgold. The question we wanted to answer was this: How much more frequent is dream recall following spontaneous awakenings out of REM sleep than those that experimentally interrupt REM sleep? The answer was seven times more frequent! All of the subjects, including me, were asked to wear the Nightcap for 10 consecutive nights and, on each of those nights, to report any mental experience that they could recall upon awakening in a hand-held tape recorder time-locked to the Nightcap. Using this protocol we could later assign the conscious states described to a physiologically defined brain state.

The Nightcap is relatively unobtrusive. Unobtrusive is, of course, relative to the massively obtrusive sleep lab gear. The subject has only to remember to put on the Nightcap and to activate its data-collection system before retiring for 10 successive nights. No big deal, right? But it's still something you might easily forget, especially as putting on the

Nightcap also commits you to recounting your experience after each awakening. Like many older people (I was 58 at the time of the study), I regularly have between two and six awakenings per night. Experience has taught me to awaken just enough to fulfill my social and physiological obligations: to keep my bed dry by going to the bathroom to urinate. I can do this now without missing a beat of sleep. But as a study subject, I now needed also to become awake enough to dictate a coherent report.

I was always a pretty good dream recaller, but with the Nightcap on my head and a tape recorder in my hand I surpassed all my previous naturalistic dream documentation. A particularly mad rush of dreaming occurred after several days in the protocol when, I suppose, I was both adapted to the Nightcap and relatively REM deprived. On night six, for instance, I had three spontaneous awakenings, each with vivid, abundant dream recall during what my Nightcap record showed to have been a single REM period! This means that I could dream, awaken, give a long coherent report, and go back into the same REM period, have another long dream, awaken, give another long and coherent report, go back to the same REM sleep epoch, dream still a third time, wake up, and report that one, too!

I was highly motivated to complete this protocol as planned, and the recognition that I was harvesting such abundant and ebullient dream recall easily countered the inconvenience of the physical Nightcap and the obligation to recount my subjective experience. No surprise then, that on night seven, when I had a dream and woke up, I dutifully reported my experience. Or I thought I had waked up. More properly speaking, I dreamed that I did! Because seconds later when I really did wake up, I was able to recall not only the original dream, but also the dream within the dream (the false awakening) and report both to my trusty tape recorder. Of course, my tape recorder had not been activated at all when I dreamed I was speaking into it, nor did my Nightcap record show any evidence of a true awakening at that time!

The upshot is that in dreams we can be twice fooled: fooled once into believing as the dream unfolds that we are awake; and fooled twice into believing that we have *really* waked up. The function of this double illusion is clear—it allows us to continue to sleep *and* to fulfill our social obligation. For once our dream's motive is crystal clear and, for once, the function of the dream is to protect sleep. The irony is that, in this case, the sleep that is endangered is endangered only—as far as we know—by the experiment, not by dreaming itself!

The experience of false awakening raises a host of fascinating questions.

The first, of course, is the deep philosophical conundrum regarding the validity of subjectivity. How can I be sure that, in my sleep, I actually dreamt and, in that same sleep, then dreamt that I dreamt? If subjectivity is so illusory, how can I trust it at all? How do I know that I didn't have all of these experiences during the awakening process or in a post-awakening carryover of the preceding REM physiology? How, in fact, do I know that I am awake even now? Can't it all be an illusion? This is not the place to consider these doubts in detail. Suffice it to say that the best assurance comes from physiology and from its already good correlation with subjectivity.

False awakening does not yet have a validating physiology. But we can be confident that, in time, it will. Its still dubious status is shared by lucid dreaming, the introduction of veridical waking consciousness into REM sleep. We might even call lucid dreaming false dreaming because a significant part of our brain is awake. So far we can only differentiate lucid dreaming physiologically by the occurrence of voluntary eye movements, a sign that has failed to convince many skeptics of the claim that lucid dreaming occurs in real time in REM sleep.

It seems to me, however, that both false awakening and lucid dreaming must have physiological substrates that are different from each other *and* different from normal REM sleep. How could such differences be revealed? Through scanning techniques, we can already predict what we will find in lucid dreaming: a reactivation of the frontal lobes sufficiently strong to allow self-reflective awareness and volition to correctly identify and to control dream consciousness but not so strong as to disrupt REM sleep. It is not so easy to know what to expect in the case of false awakening, but because it shares with lucid dreaming an increase in self-reflective awareness, I would guess that it too denotes frontal lobe reactivation to a higher level than normal REM but still lower than that of lucid dreaming.

It is wise to steer clear of these difficult questions, but history suggests that even if these particular hypotheses are not affirmed by further physiological study, the study will be fruitful in other unanticipated ways. In fact, one could argue that the agenda of cognitive neuroscience today must include a more concerted and scrupulous exploitation of such altered states of consciousness as lucid dreaming, false awakening, and hypnogogic and hypnopompic hallucinations. Because each of these conditions occurs under specifiable behavioral and neuromodulatory conditions, it seems warranted to acknowledge their subjective existence, take steps to magnify those subjective features that are distinctive of each, and then seek the specific neurobiological substrate at the level of the brain.

Out-of-Body Experiences

One of the most dramatic examples of dissociation is the famous (or infamous) subjective out-of-body state of consciousness. In this state, the subjects have (what I assume to be) the illusion that the mind has departed from the body but is hovering nearby enough to actually observe that body. They are facilitated by more explicit suggestions and by anesthetic drugs that by themselves predispose the brain to marginal states.

The question that I want to address is not whether or not out-of-body experiences actually occur. I have good reason to believe that they do, but I have deep doubts as to what they mean. In particular, I see them not as evidence that the mind and body are actually separable, but as evidence that the illusion of separability can be both vivid and extreme.

The first reason for granting a certain degree of naturalistic credence to out-of-body accounts is that in alert waking we normally experience consciousness as centered in our heads, and we see the rest of our body out there in space where we assume it actually is, but we do not ever directly perceive our brain, where (we assume) consciousness is somehow centered. When dreaming, moreover, about one-third of my respondents attest to losing this sense of head-centered consciousness and actually see their whole bodies—and selves—acting as third parties in their dreams. I myself have never had even this variant out-of-body experience. But whatever the cause or interpretation, one-third is a high proportion of people. It suggests that the illusion of being out of one's body is not that difficult for the mind to achieve when the brain is in REM sleep.

Subjects who claim to have had full-blown, bona fide out-of-body consciousness do not say "I dreamed such and such" or "It seemed so and so." No. They report their experience as if they had been fully awake.

But we already know that this conviction can be illusory and, indeed, that it normally *is* illusory when we dream. Because dreaming is an altered state of consciousness typically characterized by the illusion that we are awake and not rarely characterized by seeing the self as a third-person participant, it stands to reason that out-of-body experiences are natural, fully illusory alterations of consciousness.

The clincher in this admittedly indirect line of argument is that because dreaming is clearly an expression of an altered state of the brain, out-of-body experiences are likely the same kind of expression. Their association with head injury, with "near-death" states of consciousness, with anesthesia, and with other hypnoid marginalia would seem to make the hypothesis of organic etiology irresistible, at least to me. Supporting this organic etiology hypothesis is the reported induction of out-of-body experiences by the NMDA-glutamate receptor–blocking drugs PCP and ketamine.

Because so much is at stake (the immortality of the soul, for starters), I can understand why the faithful will resist this line of reasoning. They take the separability of mind and body as both absolute and ultimate. For them, these evanescent perceptions of separation are mere glimpses of greater promises to come. For me, they are the false harbingers of a mind-body independence that I consider untenable. Now that I think of it, an interesting hypothesis, eminently testable, is that those people who dream of themselves in the third person are either physiologically predisposed to faith or psychologically conditioned by it! Let's find out!

Alien Abduction

My astonishment at the credulity of many fellow dreamers who deny the instruction of their didactic dream illusions is exceeded only by my amazement at my even better educated colleagues, like John Mack, who collude with their patients' inferences about the veracity of alien abduction. The critique offered here is based on the testimony of the subjects that Mack describes in his book, *Alien Abduction*. However, I believe that the illusion hypothesis will apply equally well to other cases, even those that occur outdoors in the daytime. Remember, the capacity of the brain-mind for dissociation is a natural and universal talent.

Abductees are poor souls who do not leave their bodies, they take them with them to other planets! Or more properly speaking, they are taken—

body and soul together—by the most phantasmagoric third parties imaginable: little green men, ETs, and Martians. The victims of alien abductions are packed off on space ships and flying saucers. They are often subjected to gross indecencies by their captors. All of this is already belief-defying to the max. But then, *mirabile dictu,* they are returned to earth mostly safe and sound, even if indelibly altered psychologically and sometimes feeling like physically damaged goods. What are we to make of it?

Why should I discount the veracity of these witnesses? Do I believe that they are lying or faking? Not at all. I am sure they are sincere, committed believers in their experience, as I am when it comes to my lucid dreams and my false awakenings. But this is precisely the point. The abductee who believes he or she was *really* kidnapped fails to consider the very likely possibility that his or her highly convincing (and I am willing to concede genuine) subjective experience was as illusionary as my false awakening. It is important for me to state, at the onset of my critique, that I am quite open to the hypothesis of life on other planets in other solar systems. But in evaluating purported evidence of life on other planets, scientists need to be at least as skeptical as they are regarding any other possible but as yet undocumented claims. Science is a set of conceptual and methodological safeguards against what we know to be our strong innate tendency to believe. Belief, like dreaming, is a brain propensity ready to take over at regular intervals!

Among the many compelling reasons to take seriously the illusion hypothesis are the following: in John Mack's subjects, the alleged abductions typically take place at night; the abductees are often in bed; the abduction may be engineered via spacecraft typically parked on a suburban lawn, but no one else sees it. More telling still is the fact that many abductees are taken away while their spouse or significant other remains asleep and never notices their absence. They are then returned to their beds, where they may or may not alert their bed partners to the amazing and often vile adventures they have undergone.

When told to most people, alien abduction stories cause winks and laughter whether or not the people know anything about the mind's dependence on the brain and the striking correlation between sleep and altered states of consciousness. Why, they ask, should the aliens visit only at night? Why doesn't anyone else ever see them, photograph them, or even capture them? Where do the abductees go? Why do they come back?

How can it all happen so fast? And how in the world can we account for all this activity without arousing the bed partner? The only answers given to these reasonable questions are unreasonable ones: the aliens are super intelligent and ultra diabolical; precisely because they are aliens they need not obey the space-time constraints of us earthlings; in fact, their undeniable reality exposes the narrowness of earthbound reasoning. Under the circumstances, all of the assumptions of science are overthrown and replaced by a more glorious supernatural reality.

The slippery slope from acceptance of the veracity of the subjectivity of these accounts to acceptance of the veracity of the objective implications of the accounts is difficult enough to understand in the patient informants. But patients are already functionally marginal in one way or another, otherwise they would not be patients! And to understand why one cannot easily overthrow delusions, try teaching yourself lucid dreaming. It's not easy, especially if you are middle aged or older, as are most abductees. And, as with all of us, there is a lot at stake—personal credibility and personal worth, among other things.

That is why it is wise for therapists and counselors to listen carefully to accounts of alien abduction and all other probably illusional alterations of consciousness. Even physician-scientists have an interest in eliciting an unguarded report, because we need to know the whole domain of altered consciousness if we are to explain it using physicalistic concepts. But it is more than unwise for any counselor, let alone a physician-scientist, to credit such accounts with objective veracity, especially when no other competing hypothesis is taken seriously.

Psychoanalysis: Pseudoscience and Religion

It is precisely this problem, the unequivocal embrace of a speculative theory, that has held psychiatry in thrall during the century past. And, sad to say, Freudian psychoanalysis is at the root of a now popular faith that approaches religious proportions. Poor old Sigmund Freud. Through unbridled ambition and severance of ties to brain research, the confirmed atheist created an international religion. By posing as an alternative for post-graduate education in psychiatric science, psychoanalysis sets the stage for uncritical belief in a host of new-age fantasies, including claims of alien abduction.

To understand why Freud must now be turning over in his grave, we need only recall the famous incident of the spirit bookcase that led to his falling out with Carl Jung. When Jung, during a conversation between the two in Vienna, heard an unexplained noise, he proposed to Freud that his bookcase had been moved by an unseen hand! That was all Freud needed to begin the systematic expulsion of his rival. Of course, Freud had other reasons to want Jung out. Jung was sure that Freud had overemphasized sexuality, a point that even diehard Freudians now must cede to Jung! But by being himself uncritical about the causes of mental phenomena and by favoring improbable and unprovable hypotheses over simpler ones, Jung left himself open to dismissal by Freud. For his part, Jung was convinced that Freud was not only wrong in certain aspects of his psychological theory, but that Freud was altogether too materialistic in his rejection of spirituality and religious belief. It is thus no surprise that whereas many scientists prefer Freud, most humanists prefer Jung.

Like their modern day psychoanalytic counterparts, both Freud and Jung were remiss in overlooking alternative methods of studying dreams, the psychological phenomenon that formed the bedrock of their theories. Neither ever resorted to the direct observation of sleep or to the collection of dream reports in real time, and neither ever considered any neurological hypothesis about the origin and nature of dreams to be worthy of serious attention. On the contrary, Freud fiercely denounced the notion that sleep-related changes in brain physiology were responsible for the hallucinosis, the delusional belief, and the bizarre cognition of dreams, a theory very specifically articulated by physiologically oriented psychologists like Wilhelm Wundt. This is particularly strange given Freud's thorough training in neurology. Jung, the son of a Protestant pastor, fully recognized the spiritual inclinations and need for belief of human beings, and did not pretend to be scientific in his embrace of mysticism.

But what about the brain? In the first half of the twentieth century, while psychoanalysis became celebrated as a worldwide cult, neurobiology was setting its roots deep in the soil that Freud abandoned. By midcentury it was readying itself even to expose the brain mechanisms of consciousness and unconsciousness and of substrates of consciousness like dreaming. Thus Freud and Jung could be excused for not understanding that they were neglecting a promising but then underdeveloped science. Modern psychoanalysts who credit the veracity of visits by extraterrestrials have no such escape.

By the time that John Mack published his book *Alien Abduction,* sleep research was not only clearly established, it was mature enough to provide powerful, credible alternative explanations for many of the fascinating conscious experiences that occur on the margins of sleep. In fact, John Mack is also the author of an earlier book, entitled *Children's Dreams and Nightmares,* which, even as it expresses the author's psychoanalytic preferences, also reflects his awareness of modern sleep and dream science.

When all is said and done, we are forced to recognize, with Carl Jung and William James, the irresistible impulse even of highly educated scholars to believe in the witness of those reporting encounters with other worlds. Many people, including even some distinguished professors of psychiatry, are simply unwilling to settle for this world (as against others), this life (as against immortality), and this brain (as against a supernatural spirit).

In the spirit of toleration fostered so well by William James, let us admit that belief is a universal aspect of man. As such, its claims must not be dismissed out of hand. At the same time, it is crucial for cognitive neuroscientists to show, as I have tried to do here, that the brain is easily bamboozled, especially in sleep and at its margins, but also, of course, in waking. That is why a leading hypothesis advanced in explaining unusual states of consciousness must be unusual states of brain. Of course, the universally shared tendency to believe is also subject to co-option by social forces, including institutions that can both support and inculcate faith in improbable agencies.

To help the reader understand the reasons for this emphasis on the brain, we now turn our attention to two specific disorders of sleep and dreaming that illustrate, respectively, a genetically determined predisposition to experience dreamlike consciousness in waking (narcolepsy) and an acquired tendency to express dream behavior in sleep (REM sleep behavior disorder). The existence of these clear abnormalities emphasizes what we have learned earlier in the chapter about the normal difficulty we have in containing dreaming to consciousness within sleep.

Narcolepsy

One of my first narcoleptic patients had been treated by a psychoanalytically inclined psychiatrist who attributed one of her symptoms, cataplexy, to anxiety about sex. Not that she wasn't anxious about sex—in the early 1950s every "nice" girl *was* anxious about sex. If you weren't anxious about sex, you weren't a nice girl! This logic is a little bit like the European Witch Trials, when those who perished when held under water were considered innocent because they had insufficient witch power to be saved, while those who survived were obviously strongly possessed and needed to be dunked again. If you were not anxious about sex in the 1950s, you were obviously a prostitute.

But not many of the nice girls that I knew expressed their anxiety by becoming paralyzed during orgasm! And they didn't suddenly fall asleep at dinner parties, nor did they fall to the floor when they heard a joke, even if it was an off-color joke! We're not talking about convulsive laughter. We're talking about muscle atonia. In explaining these symptoms, too, the psychoanalysts resorted to their fail-safe logic: guilty of repressed sexual impulses and/or guilt about same and no way to prove your innocence! Worse than that, no alternative hypothesis need be considered!

The alternative hypothesis and the hypothesis of my choice, that of neurogenesis rather than psychogenesis, *should* have been considered. Why? Because the muscle atonia associated with narcoleptic cataplexy is caused by an active inhibition that is detectable with a reflex hammer, one of the useful medical instruments that the psychoanalysts threw away when they took off their white coats and jettisoned experimental science for the pseudo-science of sexual symbol decoding. And there were other strong clues: narcoleptic patients complained of dreaming at sleep onset, whereas Freud asserted that dreaming only occurred in the instant before awakening. The way out of this is to say, "Sure, you see the repressed sexuality and related guilt are so strong as to break through the minute that the ego releases its hold on the unconscious when you fall asleep."

Of course, the unwitting analysts didn't know about REM sleep in the early 1950s. No one did. But this same kind of ad hoc, circular reasoning persisted for at least twenty years after 1953, when REM sleep was discovered and narcolepsy was immediately recognized as an abnormal intensification of REM physiology, all of whose symptoms could be explained neurodynamically. Besides the difficulty maintaining alertness and postural muscle tone during waking (because the cholinergic REM-on system was unusually strong and the aminergic REM-off system unusually weak), narcoleptic patients had an exaggerated tendency to sleep onset imagery (hypnagogic hallucinations), to post-awakening persistent dream imagery (hypnopompic hallucinations), and to sleep paralysis (REM sleep atonia extended into waking).

To appreciate just how powerful an erroneous speculation theory can be, *all* of these symptoms were rationalized as instinct and emotion gone wild! We now know that REM sleep, the culprit in narcolepsy, *is* instinct and emotion gone wild, but not in a Freudian sense. The instinct in question is survival, not procreation, and the emotion in question is fear, not pleasure. In REM sleep, fear is the natural response to amygdala activation. It is reflexively triggered as circuits essential to survival are cholinergically stimulated and glutamatergically mediated. The survival function of this reflex is clear: sense danger, run away. Now this *is* defense. But not in the psychoanalytic sense!

When the narcoleptic patient, for whatever reason, trips his or her startle circuit, the tendency is great to trigger REM, the off-line proxy of escape behavior. Of course, triggering REM under *these* circumstances is evolutionarily *mal*adaptive (as well as socially inconvenient!). Some might think that cataplexy is some variant of the "freeze" response that enables animals both to escape detection and to evaluate their options in the face of predator, but it is certainly not a good idea for a gazelle to fall to the ground in front of a hungry lion. Narcoleptic gazelles are goners, and their genes are goners too. They are lions' lunch. The neurodynamics of narcolepsy are represented in figure 8.2.

So how have humans with narcolepsy managed to survive and continue to pass their genes for this unfortunate tendency along to their offspring? One answer is that despite their alleged sexual phobias and their orgasmic cataplexy, narcoleptic men and women to manage to copulate and to reproduce successfully! The second answer is ecological. Most of us are not exposed to leonine predators. Even a narcoleptic caveman or cavewoman may have survived to reproductive age by protective devices such as the cave itself, parents, siblings, and mates. And if a modern narcoleptic were to fall down limp during an armed robbery, would the robber be more—or less—likely to off his victim?

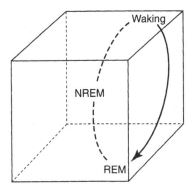

Figure 8.2
In narcolepsy, subjects may reverse the normal trajectory as shown in figure 2.8 and enter REM directly from waking at both nocturnal sleep onset and during daytime sleep attacks. This propensity is caused by a combination of relatively weak aminergic drive and reciprocally intensified cholinergic drive, which result in a marked lowering of the wake-REM threshold.

But the best answer to the survival question is pharmacological treatment, because it provides significant symptom relief. Pharmacological treatment is also the best answer because it closes the scientific circle so tightly and neatly. The drugs that work are those that promote waking and demote REM sleep. They promote waking by potentiating the biogenic amines that are necessary to maintain alertness. Significantly, in the case of narcolepsy, these clearly include dopamine, norepinephrine, and serotonin. By promoting the biogenic amines these drugs also indirectly demote REM. Some of the very best antinarcoleptic drugs also directly demote REM, via their anticholinergic actions.

The narcolepsy story is important not only because it explains the sleep disorder itself, but because we can use it to begin to understand the normal dynamics of brain state transitions. The narcolepsy story supports the general hypothesis that state margins are fuzzy, not sharp; ragged, not smooth; and mushy, not crisp. State transitions need finite amounts of time to be fully accomplished. Because so many subsystems of the brain participate it is not surprising that one (or two) should lag behind (or lead) the rest. The net result is that we can be in two states at once: waking *and* dreaming.

Extrapolating from the narcolepsy story and from the well-known neurophysiology of REM sleep we can, moreover, begin to construct a general theory of conscious state alteration that specifies the behavioral and biochemical conditions under which they are likely to occur. The general hypothesis that emerges also integrates a regional view of the brain with the neuromodulatory approach. Because this integrated model incorporates both relatively automatic emotional and instinct-driven forces with relatively deliberate, volitional, and personally meaningful motives, it not only cuts across levels of neurobiolgical analysis, but engages psychology in a clinically meaningful way.

No doubt the patient with narcolepsy can benefit from psychotherapy combined with drug treatment. All patients with such seriously disabling symptoms need a supportive, didactic, and exploratory dialogue with a concerned and knowledgeable professional, preferably the same person who is managing the pharmacological treatment. But a psychotherapy that is scientifically responsible will never assume, or even suggest, that the symptoms themselves are psychogenic, the expression of covert motives, or the acting out of unconscious wishes. The narcolepsy story shows clearly how easily mistaken and misguided the hermeneutic (or symbolic) approach can be and how dangerous was the demedicalization of psychiatry. Separating psychiatry and neurology is as foolish as separating mind from brain. "What God has joined together let no man put asunder" is the priestly admonition to wedding congregations. Substitute "Nature" for "God," and we could say the same to the vast congregation of psychologists who yearn for the scientific legitimacy of a proper marriage of mind and brain!

The REM Sleep Behavior Disorder

Mea culpa! Having scolded the psychoanalysts for their egregious folly in misinterpreting narcolepsy and dreaming, I now admit my own guilt of a similar misinterpretation. It took me longer than I like to admit to recognize that patients who clearly described the behavioral expression of their dreams were trying to help me discover a new clinical condition, the REM sleep behavior disorder, and not simply misconstruing common, garden variety somnambulism. That this recognition came from the application of sleep lab technology is doubly embarrassing. Knowing how surprising and informative this technique can be, I should have been the first to use it.

There are two sharp twists in this story. The first is the explosion of folk psychology myths about sleepwalking, such as that sleepwalkers were enacting their dreams—they are not—or that it is dangerous to wake up a sleepwalker. It may be impossible, but it is *not* dangerous. Both myths founder on the shoals of sleep physiology. Sleepwalkers, who are usually children or adolescents, are having trouble rising from the depths of slow wave or NREM sleep. As they walk they sleep.

Sleepwalkers demonstrate still another fuzzy boundary: they are motorically awake but cognitively (read consciously) asleep. This dissociation can be objectified by sleep lab techniques that have demonstrated that high voltage, slow waves can emanate from the thalamocortical system during the sleepwalking episode. Such conscious mental activity may be present in confused, low-level intentionality like "I need to go to the bathroom," but where the bathroom is and what to do when I get there is not at all clear! This is not dreaming. And although it is possible that the sleepwalker can be guided to the bathroom (and induced to urinate there rather than in the flower garden) he or she may never fully wake up at all, nor have any recollection of the nocturnal wanderings the next morning.

Other dissociations are the altered states of consciousness seen in hypnosis and hysteria that have been likened to sleepwalking. The word "somnambulism" denotes not only sleepwalking per se, it also denotes those hypnotic trance states that impose a kind of sleepiness on susceptible subjects during waking. For Pierre Janet (and for Charcot, Freud, and the rest), this was the very essence of dissociation. The psychoanalytic model ascribed the same repressed libidinal wishes to the hypnotic somnambulist that it found to be the root cause of all dreaming. The fact of the matter is that *any* coordinated behavior is likely to invite the ascription of motive. If the subject is unconscious or nonconscious, then the motive must be unconscious too.

But do all such automatisms constitute—or denote—motives? Impulsive motion, yes. But psychological motive, I'm not so sure. Now I need to get back to my confession.

Because sleepwalking does not occur in REM sleep and because REM sleep is defined, in part, by inhibition of postural muscle tone and by the absence of any but the smallest inconsequential movements, I made the mistake of assuming that dreams could never be enacted. This was foolish of me. In the first place, some dreaming occurs outside of REM. Further-more, the motor inhibition of REM is only partial, not absolute. The countervailing motor excitation may normally be low enough to be quelled but might increase enough to overcome the inhibition. We see this opposition in the related condition of sleeptalking. When a subject cries out in response to dream anxiety he supposes his communication is articulate but his bed partner often hears only muffled vocalization. More articulate sleeptalking may not be associated with dreaming at all. Despite being aware of these facts, I continued to miss the distinction between sleepwalking and dreamwalking for about four years!

Several patients and their observant spouses told me gripping tales of dream enactment. Dreaming that he is a star setback, one patient sud-denly gets up, runs across room, and collides with the dresser. Dreaming that he is driving on a perilously curving road and needs to make a sharp left turn, a patient who is supine suddenly flings his left arm in a 180 degree arch and swats his wife. Dreaming that he is operating to remove a tumor deep in the third ventricle, a neurosurgeon patient makes elaborate movements with his outstretched hands and issues clearly articulated ver-bal orders to hallucinatory assistants to "grab that retractor," "give me a kelly clamp."

How could I have been so stupid for so long? All of these patients were older men. All of them were easily aroused from their altered states of consciousness. And all of them gave detailed reports of subjective dream-ing that perfectly matched their movements. They could not have been run of the mill somnambulists. It was the neurosurgeon that woke me up because he, like many narcoleptic patients, had his attacks during the daytime, and when he did, he was observably asleep with rapid eye move-ments but without atonia! Another day, another dissociation. By the time we are finished we will have seen them all!

When we recorded the neurosurgeon's sleep, the scales finally fell from my eyes. He could not possibly have been a sleepwalker because he did not have one single slow wave (or spindle) all night long! Nothing but REM—but all of his REM was without muscle atonia! The neurosur-geon dreamed continuously of operating, acting out each surgical sce-nario with his hands! Obviously, this is *not* normal REM, and it is *not* normal dreaming. But it is sleep with rapid eye (and hand) movements, and the associated state of consciousness is fully hallucinating if not intrinsically bizarre! So how was *this* dissociation affected? How had the atonia so normally typical of REM been subtracted? Could that subtraction have anything to do with what was added, namely the excessive REM pressure that caused him to have dream attacks by day and to dream all night?

Bells began to ring in my head! I had seen REM sleep without atonia before. It was in Michel Jouvet's lab in the early 1960s, when he and his team were trying to selectively damage the locus coeruleus, which, they mistakenly believed, actively commanded REM. This meant that my neurosurgeon patient probably had a disease process affecting his brain stem, a possibility that had already been raised by his earlier symptoms of sleeplessness and difficulty with balance and coordination.

But Jouvet's cats had normal slow wave sleep and only showed their stereotyped attack and defense behaviors during otherwise normal REM periods, not during waking, and not all night long. So the neurosurgeon's brainstem disease process could not be the same as Jouvet's experimental destruction. No. If it involved destruction then as it ultimately and fatally did, it also involved stimulation—intense, preemptive stimulation of the REM sleep generator circuits projecting to the upper brain. It is reasonable to speculate that this abnormal excitation selectively activated the human equivalent of the PGO generator zone in the lateral pons where cholinergic neurons abound and where exogenous cholinergic stimulation also gives prolonged and preemptive REM sleep enhancement.

Neurodynamic Dysfunction and Neurological Disease

The REM sleep behavior disorder has carried us across the border between functional sleep disorders associated with easily reversible alterations in consciousness to structural disease of the brain associated with irreversible alterations in consciousness, leading to its ultimate loss in coma and death. Whether that border—like the border between the normal states of consciousness—is fuzzy or sharp, ragged or smooth, continuous or discontinuous, remains to be seen, but one thing is clear: the border between the functional and the structural can be crossed and when it is, the states of consciousness are permanently altered. They also vividly instruct us to keep our eyes open for new and unexpected discoveries and our minds open for new and surprising concepts.

One unexpected observation, which I will discuss in chapter 10, is that some SSRI drugs that potentiate the serotonin system in favor of enhanced mood in depression cause disturbingly long-lasting alterations in REM sleep physiology, and these alterations sometimes cross the border into the REM sleep behavior disorder.

Why the SSRIs should disorganize sleep in the way that they do is not yet clear. Serotonin inhibits REM sleep and participates in the control of eye movement in waking, too. One might therefore suppose that enhancing serotonin would suppress eye movements, but instead they appear in super-abundance during (so-called) non-REM sleep, as well as in REM. I say so-called because there are, in fact, *some* eye movements in that sleep phase that is supposed not to have any! But the SSRIs cause them to be continuous and—interestingly—cause continuous dreaming, too. These signs, which occur early in SSRI treatment, are still another manifestation of dissociation, and imply already abnormal effects of the drug on the motor control mechanisms of sleep that are akin to the RBD syndrome into which they may merge after months of SSRI use. The upshot, stated strongly for emphasis, is that the treatment of one disease (depression) may cause another (RBD).

As I write, this important frontier is just beginning to be explored and what I say about it should be taken as tentative hypothesizing, but I want to make the central hypothesis crystal clear: artificial alteration of the neuromodulatory systems that control consciousness can produce potent changes, some desirable and some decidedly undesirable. This means that a scrupulous and conservative cost-benefit analysis needs to be undertaken during the next few years, when we can expect the use of these agents to peak and their long-term effects to become more obvious.

9

Brain Dysfunctions that Alter Consciousness

The dependence of consciousness upon brain state has always been most clearly shown by the deficits and distortions associated with structural and functional neurological disease. Damage to the brain, caused by trauma or vascular insufficiency, can result in the loss of neurons essential to the direct maintenance of consciousness, leading to coma; brain damage can also alter consciousness by disconnecting brain regions whose integration is necessary to the normal subjective experiences of conscious state change. Contrastingly, if the neurons become hyperexcitable—as they certainly do in epilepsy and most probably do in some drug withdrawal states—then some aspects of consciousness may become exaggerated at the expense of others. Among the most interesting examples are the "dreamy states" associated with temporal lobe seizures.

When both the effects of brain destruction and the effects of brain overactivity are localized to the same region—and cause reciprocal effects—they give added credence to the hypothesis of causality. That is to say, the region in question really is essential to the function under investigation. Either intervention, taken alone, can be misleading because lesions interrupt pathways linking essential structures and stimulation effects can be broadcast in the brain via those linking pathways. In fact, the cognitive neuroscience literature is a veritable graveyard of theories that were based on an exclusive reliance on only one method of investigation.

Research on the alterations in consciousness caused by sleep has recently been greatly augmented by two sources of evidence that we can scrutinize for instances of complementary enhancement and disruption of function. They are studies of selective brain activation utilizing PET and fMRI neuroimaging techniques, already mentioned in chapters 6 and 7, and the close questioning regarding dreaming of patients who have suffered well-localized brain damage due to strokes. It is the goal of this chapter to review these findings critically and to integrate their implications with the findings of basic research at the cellular and molecular level in animals. By adding the basic neurobiology data to the mix I hope to achieve an even stronger criterion of confidence to that provided by the complementary neuroimaging and brain lesion findings.

Let me explain by introducing a model of conscious state control that is at once global and distributed but involves highly specific and well-localized brain mechanisms. This model provides a framework for discussing the brain lesion and stimulation data. Considering consciousness and its normal vicissitudes as we have defined and discussed them with special reference to waking and dreaming, now we need to answer the following questions:

• Where does the conscious experience actually arise? Few neurocognitivists doubt that the answer is the forebrain, and most would now posit the participation of widely distributed but interconnected circuits in the neocortex and in subcortical centers like the basal ganglia and limbic structures.

• Under what circumstances does conscious experience arise in the forebrain? Few neuroscientists now doubt that the distributed and interconnected cortical circuits that are the physical substrate of conscious experience need to be synchronously activated, probably via the widely distributed thalamocortical system.

• What is the source of the activation of the thalamocortical system and the distributed forebrain circuits underlying consciousness? Few neuroscientists now doubt that the brainstem reticular formation, and especially its pontine-mesencephalic and diencephalic components, regulate the cortex via its interaction with the thalamocortical system.

The three preceding questions and answers apply to any state of consciousness, to dreaming as well as waking, as long as that state of consciousness achieves an integrated awareness of the world (be it real or fictive), the body (be it connected or disconnected), and the self (be it fully or only partially accurate). In every case, there is complementary evidence to support these hypotheses:

• The contention that consciousness actually arises in the forebrain is confirmed by its absence in anencephalic children and by the possibility of restoring consciousness by chemical stimulation of the modulatory systems when the brain stem is intact in some cases of coma or unresponsiveness.

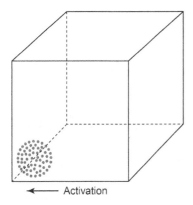

← Activation

Figure 9.1
Coma. Consciousness is impossible in coma because the activation level is low, aminergic drive is down, and the sensorimotor gates are closed. Thus the coma domain is in the left front corner of the state space. There are, of course, many variations on the theme of coma, such as coma vigil and locked-in syndrome, which would occupy different positions of the state space.

• The contention that the thalamocortical system is essential to the synchronous activation of the forebrain and hence to consciousness is supported by the loss of consciousness in subjects with disease destruction of the thalamus and by the capacity to restore consciousness by activating the thalamocortical system if that system (and of course, the cortex) is intact. The case of Karen Ann Quinlan is well known: her profound coma was caused by a very small, restricted thalamic lesion and was irreversible because the thalamocortical system could not be activated by any known means.

• The critical role of the brain stem in the synchronous activation of the distributed forebrain circuits via thalamocortical activation is strongly evidenced by the fact that the most devastating and irreversible impairments of consciousness occur as deep and often irreversible comas following brainstem trauma or stroke. If the brain stem is only functionally impaired, as by the loss of one or more of its chemical modulators, then consciousness can be restored if that chemical function is simulated. The famous example of "awakening" following the correction of dopamine deficiency in severely damaged postencephalitic Parkinsonism illustrates this point The neurodynamics of coma are represented in figure 9.1.

So far we have emphasized those structures and functions essential to consciousness of any kind, be it waking or dreaming. This sets the stage for the more difficult question as to how we can differentiate those two kinds of consciousness. In discussing the basic neurobiology in chapter 6, and outlining the AIM model in chapter 7, I have already provided detailed data regarding the questions I now pose and again answer in summary form here.

• What accounts for the fact that dreaming consciousness occurs during sleep? In other words, why doesn't the activation of the thalamocortical system during REM result in awakening? The most pertinent answer to this question is that the input-output gates are closed by inhibitory deactivation of sensory input channels and motor output portals. In this view, dreaming is simply an off-line variant of waking consciousness. But that is not the case. Dreaming is distinctly different from waking in many important ways.

• What causes the distinctive, intrinsic differences between waking and dreaming consciousness? There are two answers to this question. The first is that the neuromodulatory input from the pontine brain stem to the cortex is altered with a marked weakening of noradrenergic and serotonergic influence and a marked enhancement of cholinergic influence (at least at the level of the pons, midbrain, hypothalamus, and thalamus). The second answer is the set of differences in regional activation with intensification of blood flow in the limbic subcortex (e.g., amygdala), the parahippocampal and anterior cingulate cortices, the basal ganglia, the basal forebrain, and the parietal operculum, and with deficient blood flow to the dorsolateral prefrontal cortex. It remains to be seen if these two answers are independent or interdependent.

What evidence exists to support or inform these hypotheses?

With respect to the input-output gating issue, we know from recording studies in humans that sensory thresholds to arousal are higher in REM than in stage II, though not as high as in stages III–IV of NREM sleep. The diminution, during human REM sleep, of the amplitude of the H-reflex, measured as the magnitude of muscle twitch response to electrical stimulation of the homologous sensory nerve, shows that motor output is actively blocked. In chapter 8 we saw that the intensification of REM sleep mediating circuits that occurs in narcolepsy can potentiate the descending muscle tone inhibition (in sleep paralysis and in cataplexy) at the same time that the internal circuits mediating the fictive percepts of dreaming are intensified by excitatory stimuli of brainstem origin. We have also seen that damage to the brain stem, as in early Parkinsonism, can result in a loss of the ability to contain the fictive movement of REM sleep wake pattern activation.

With respect to the possible contribution of differential neuromodulation to the cognitive differences between sleeping and waking, we unfortunately have as yet very little direct evidence in humans. The indirect evidence constitutes the balance of this book. The psychopharmacological data from both medical and recreational drug sources generally supports the hypothesis, but there are many important exceptions that constitute problems for this aspect of the model. Two complementary facts at this chemical level of analysis strengthen the model:

• The first is that the activity of chemically specific cell groups correlates more strongly than any other brain measure with REM sleep vs. waking neurophysiology in animals (and hence, by implication, with dreaming vs. waking consciousness in humans).

• The second is that the most potent means of experimentally driving waking consciousness in the direction of dream consciousness in humans is to introduce drugs that directly interact with the specific chemical neuromodulators that change naturally in the wake to dream consciousness alterations.

An Alternative Model of Dreaming

Since the activation synthesis hypothesis of dreaming was first enunciated in 1977, critics have voiced the concern that it overemphasized the dependence of dreaming on REM sleep. Dreaming can occur in the absence of REM, especially at sleep onset and during Stage II sleep in the early morning hours prior to awakening. Such dissociations of dreaming from REM sleep indicate that the forebrain could enter physiological states capable of engendering dream consciousness without the brain stem's involvement. It was therefore further proposed that the forebrain mechanisms of dreaming were autonomous of brainstem influence and that REM sleep physiology was incidental to dreaming.

With respect to the integrated model proposed here, the forebrain-activation alternative to AIM also emphasized changes in activation but postulated a shift toward intrinsic cortico-cortical inputs as the main source of endogenous stimulation. The forebrain activation model was therefore not related either to input-output gating in the periphery or to the changes in the rates of aminergic-cholinergic neuromodulation of the forebrain. A slight change in activation was all that was needed to produce the shift from waking to dreaming consciousness, and a change in forebrain activation was thus necessary and sufficient to produce dreaming.

Proponents of the forebrain activation hypothesis often advocated the related view that consciousness was always more or less dreamlike. Even waking could support dreamlike mentation, as the common occurrence of fantasy and of daydreaming attested. Changing the environmental stimulus level by putting a subject at rest in a darkened room was enough to tip the balance of cortical activation in the direction of intrinsic cortico-cortical stimuli and to thus foster the production of mental experiences formally indistinguishable from dreaming. Sleep was seen as an only incidental step along a continuum of consciousness. For many psychologists, no significant differences in conscious state existed between REM and NREM sleep. This alternative model has great appeal to cognitive scientists who want to model activation without coming to grips with its physiologically complex and manifold underpinnings, and to psychologists who wish to create a science of dreams that is independent of physiology. In the latter category are many latter-day Freudians interested in hermeneutic approaches to mental life and to dream interpretive schemata that are immune to criticisms based upon neurophysiology.

I consider it to be a matter of fact that consciousness is a continuum of states, that aspects of two or more sometimes distinct states can co-exist, that consciousness can be dreamlike even in waking, and that it is likely to be more so at sleep onset. I also know that dreaming can occur in light sleep in the early morning. It thus seems to me quite reasonable to propose that we can explain many of these facts by changes in the level and distribution of activation in the forebrain, and that one forebrain site can become an input source for another.

But all of these allowances do not in any way diminish the scientific value of studying REM physiology and relating it to dreaming, because the optimal conditions for dreaming are achieved in REM sleep and the study of REM sleep is therefore the most powerful approach to understanding the physiology of dreaming. The three-dimensional AIM model based on that study thus provides the richest framework for understanding dreaming and other altered states of consciousness.

I therefore consider the alternative model to be perfectly reasonable as far as it goes, but assert that it does not go far enough. I further believe that its important claims can easily be integrated into the new

AIM version of activation synthesis. The original activation synthesis model is shown in figure 9.2, and its updating in AIM is presented in figure 9.3.

Important technical arguments regarding the definition and measurement of the many aspects of consciousness and brain physiology that characterize the full spectrum of conscious states from alert waking through dreamy drowsiness and light sleep to full blown, sustained REM sleep dreaming need to be confirmed and settled before a consensus can be reached—and given the strength of many of the positions taken in these arguments, consensus may never be possible. The reader who is interested in the details of this argument may wish to consult our target article entitled "Dreaming and the Brain," the commentaries elicited by it, and our response to those commentaries, entitled "Dream Science 2000," all of which were published together in the open, peer-commentary journal, *Behavioral and Brain Sciences* in December 2000.

The Effects of Brain Lesions on Dreaming in Humans

A classic method of human neuropsychology is to investigate the changes in function that are associated with damage to the brain. For example, the importance of the hippocampal formation of the temporal lobe to declarative or explicit memory acquisition was established by testing the memory capacity of subjects whose hippocampal formations had been surgically disconnected for other medical reasons. Much of what we know about language comes from the study of patients with stroke damage to language areas in the temporal and frontal cortex.

Perhaps one reason that it took so long for neuropsychologists to investigate dreaming after stroke damage to the brain is that there are no tests for dreaming. One simply asks, "Did you notice any change in your dreams after your stroke?" It's too easy! But because of the arbitrary division of psychiatry and neurology it was also too difficult for either group to pose the question. Neurologists who treated stroke patients weren't supposed to talk about dreams and psychiatrists who were obliged to talk about dreams didn't see stroke patients! Furthermore, many psychiatrists don't make mental status exams, and even if they had heard that some patients stopped dreaming after their strokes, they would have interpreted the symptom as unbridled repression!

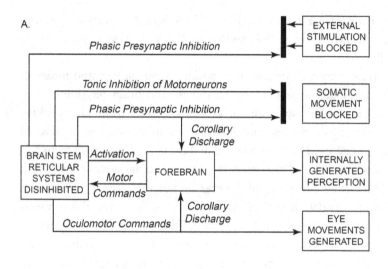

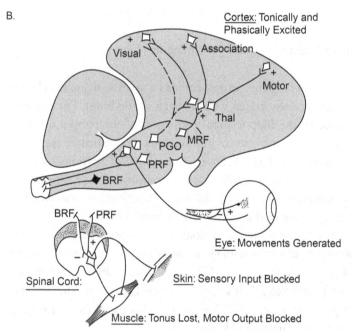

Figure 9.2
Activation-synthesis model. (A) Systems model. (B) Wiring diagram. As a result of
disinhibition caused by cessation of aminergic neuronal firing, brainstem reticular
systems autoactivate. Their outputs have effects including depolarization of afferent terminals causing phasic presynaptic inhibition and blockade of external stimuli, especially during the bursts of REM, and postsynaptic hyperpolarization

And, indeed, although the question *is* easy to ask, the answer is *not* easy to interpret. Suppose the patient says that he stopped dreaming after his stroke? Should we take the answer seriously? Of course. But uncritically? Certainly not, because dream recall depends upon memory and memory is both notoriously poor for dreaming and notoriously subject to damage from stroke, especially if the damage is in or near the temporal lobes. It also seems quite likely that sleep itself would change after a stroke. If subjects slept less well, they might not so easily enter REM or other brain activation states associated with dreaming; they would wake up instead. If they slept more deeply, their recall would be impaired.

A thorough neuropsychological study would also need to include a prospective as well as a retrospective probe, and it would require the objective documentation of sleep. We could accomplish this goal in a sleep lab, hospital room, or home setting where sleep was objectively monitored and awakenings performed in REM and NREM sleep at protocol-determined times of night. We would also want to know if mental activity other than dreaming was associated with poststroke sleep. Further, because many of the patients could be expected to recover cerebral function and dreaming, the time course of the evolution of these features should also be documented.

This sets the stage for such studies as those reported in the recent book by Mark Solms, a neuropsychologist working in London, on the reports of a discontinuation of dreaming in a group of 334 patients who were questioned by the author after suffering cerebral damage such as strokes. Despite the many shortcomings of the study, the results are of capital importance because they provide preliminary evidence that is complementary to the PET scan studies performed simultaneously by others,

causing tonic inhibition of motorneurons that effectively counteract concomitant motor commands so that somatic movement is blocked. Only the oculomotor commands are read out as eye movements because these motorneurons are not inhibited. The forebrain, activated by the reticular formation and also aminergically disinhibited, receives efferent copy or corollary discharge information about somatic motor and oculomotor commands from which it may synthesize such internally generated perceptions as visual imagery and the sensation of movement, both of which typify dream mentation. The forebrain may, in turn, generate its own motor commands that help to perpetuate the process via positive feedback to the reticular formation. (From Hobson, 1988)

Activation

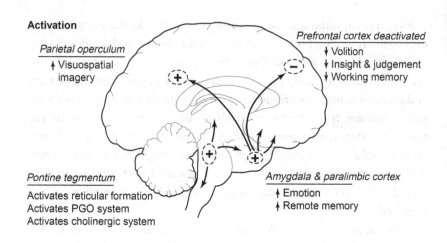

Parietal operculum
↑ Visuospatial
  imagery

Prefrontal cortex deactivated
↓ Volition
↓ Insight & judgement
↓ Working memory

Pontine tegmentum
Activates reticular formation
Activates PGO system
Activates cholinergic system

Amygdala & paralimbic cortex
↑ Emotion
↑ Remote memory

Input Source

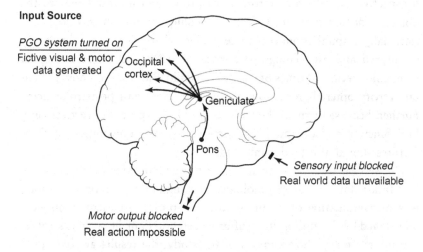

PGO system turned on
Fictive visual & motor
  data generated

Occipital
cortex

Geniculate

Pons

Sensory input blocked
Real world data unavailable

Motor output blocked
Real action impossible

Modulation

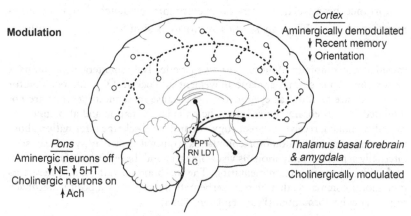

Cortex
Aminergically demodulated
↓ Recent memory
↓ Orientation

Pons
Aminergic neurons off
↓ NE, ↓ 5HT
Cholinergic neurons on
↑ Ach

PPT
RN LDT
LC

*Thalamus basal forebrain
& amygdala*

Cholinergically modulated

unbeknownst to Solms. The PET results are summarized in figure 9.4 and compared with the brain lesion effects in table 9.1.

The two regions whose damage caused patients to report a complete cessation of dreaming were the supramarginal gyrus (on the cortical surface) and the mediobasal forebrain (in the depths of the brain). Both of these areas are among the relatively few brain regions that imaging techniques have revealed to receive increases in blood flow during REM sleep. Note well that insofar as the strength of Solms's findings depends upon a reciprocity with the PET findings, it is only in REM sleep and not in NREM that these areas are activated. Hence, we cannot yet attribute any dreaming that occurs in NREM sleep to the activation of these areas.

The *supramarginal gyrus* is at the cortical junction of visual and spatial processing regions. It is situated between the occipital and temporal regions, the interconnections of which pass through the area. Before Solms' work was published, several other groups had suggested that stroke damage to the supramarginal gyrus impaired dreaming. Cristiano Violani and Fabrizio Doricchi came to this conclusion based on a literature review of neurological cases, most of them isolated, where a loss of dreaming was reported. Martha Farah and Mark Greenberg independently described a set of patients with the same syndrome, and the Pisa neurological group led by Drs. Muri and Muratorri found that the supramarginal gyrus over the region was at the center of their maps of cortical damage by stroke causing a loss of dreaming.

This concatenation of evidence leads us to take the claim that dreaming depends upon the integrity of the supramarginal gyrus very seriously indeed. What are we to make of the finding? We have long known that the supramarginal gyrus plays an important role in visuospatial integration. Through its intrinsic cellular activity and via its interconnections with the visual, auditory, and somatosensory processing centers situated all

---

Figure 9.3
AIM. Physiological signs and regional brain mechanisms of REM sleep dreaming separated into activation (A), input source (I), and modulation (M) functional components of the AIM model. Dynamic changes in A, I, and M during REM sleep dreaming are noted adjacent to each figure. Note that these are highly schematized depictions that illustrate global processes and do not attempt to comprehensively detail all the brain structures and their interactions that may be involved in REM sleep dreaming.

A. **Waking**

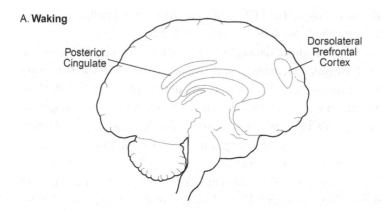

B. **NREM Sleep (cf waking)**

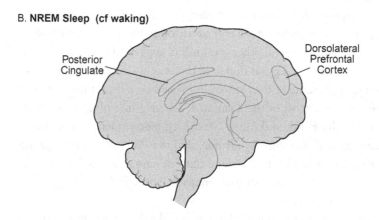

C. **REM (cf waking)**

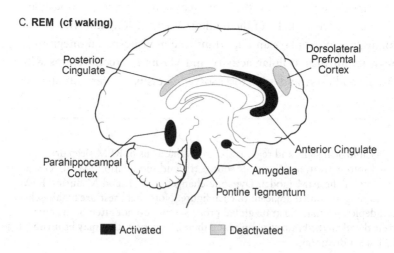

Table 9.1
Imaging of Brain Activation in REM and the Effects of Brain Lesions on Dreaming

Region	Pet Studies on Activation in REM	Lesion Studies of Effects on Dreaming
Pontine tegmentum	↑	–
Limbic structures	↑	↓
Visual cortex	–	–
Supramarginal gyrus	↑	↓
Dorsolateral prefrontal cortex	↓	–
Mediobasal frontal cortex	↑	↓

Key: ↑, increase; ↓, decrease; –, no change.

around it, it makes a self-centered and unified three-dimensional map of the world available to us as an integral and constant component of conscious experience. Thus we perceive ourselves as agents moving through the world. This aspect of consciousness is present, remarkably strongly, in dreaming.

Close studies of dream phenomenology, from Helmholtz's early self-observations to recent formal analyses of sleep laboratory and home-based dream reports of thousands of subjects, point to the convincing illusion of movement through dream space as the perceptual essence of dream consciousness. Although it is difficult enough to imagine how such a faithful and useful percept could be created in waking when our eyes are open and we are really acting in the world—so allowing visual and proprioceptive signals to have a close correspondence to an external physical reality—it is truly mind-boggling to appreciate that exclusively internal activation of the brain can so impressively simulate this experience during dreaming.

Figure 9.4
PET results. Summary of PET study evidence of brain region activation in NREM and REM sleep. Compared to the blood flow distribution in waking (A), the global decreases observed in NREM sleep (B) suggest widespread deactivation consistent with the greatly diminished capacity for conscious experience early in the night. In REM sleep, many regions are activated above their levels in waking (solid black) while others are deactivated (shaded). These changes are consistent with the vivid perceptual and emotional character of dream consciousness and with its impoverished capacity for analytic, directed thought. (From Hobson et al., *NeuroReport 9*: R1–R14.)

Virtual reality is the name given to the computer simulation of movement through space when the features of a digitally recreated visual scene change in synchrony with a subject's head and extremity movements. This is getting pretty close to what goes on in dreams—except that there is no real movement to use as a signal source for integration with the artificial visual imagery. In the virtual reality of dreaming consciousness, *everything* is artificial, except of course the eye movement in REM. Yet, as far as we know, neither the eye movements of REM—nor those of waking—generate any feedback signals that could be used to program the virtual reality of dreams.

We are thus forced to acknowledge that the convincing sense of movement through dream space is made up from feedforward, not feedback, information. The fact that we are able to do this so well when we are completely disconnected from the world makes us aware of just how much internal environment autonomous processing may go on in waking when our subjective impression is of an exclusive reliance on data from the outside world.

The results of the PET and brain lesion studies summarized together in table 9.1 force us also to realize how much the subjective experience of dreaming is dependent upon the integrity of visuospatial integration. Subjects with stroke-induced dream deficiencies in visuospatial integration can apparently compensate for these defects in waking. They have no evident difficulty in navigating through the world. After all, the external world is really out there issuing a constant stream of data whose parameters change as a function of the very real movements that the subject can still make. But in dreaming, the visuospatial simulator is so seriously disenabled that, if we take the subjects at their word, dreaming ceases altogether. It would be interesting to test patients with loss of dreaming owing to parietal cortex strokes for the ability to visualize complex imagery with their eyes closed but awake. This skill could be impaired but go unnoticed unless a specific probe were made.

It is always dangerously easy to understand scientific facts after they have been established. We call this the power of the retrospectoscope. But this one really does make sense, especially as it fits so well with the phenomenological evidence. Still, we would like to know much, much more about these patients. Why, for example, does sleep thinking stop? Why, also, does sleep emotion stop? It should still be possible, certainly, for these patients to ruminate—even painfully—about their damaged brain-minds. And what about their ability to create visual imagery during waking? Have any of Stephen Kosslyn's ingenious tasks of visual imagery generation been used to assess handicaps in waking that may not be easily noticed by the subjects?

With respect to their sleep, are their eye movement patterns the same or different from age and sex matched normal subjects? Before we conclude that it is only the cortical damage that results in loss of dreaming, shouldn't we consider the possibility that the brain stem changes its behavior in response to the cortical lesion? The question is all the more salient because lesions of the nearby parietal cortex *do* cause peculiar eye movement patterns and are associated with peculiar changes in visual perception. In a sense, what is going on here is the logical extension of neuropsychology into the vast and fascinating domain of sleep and dreams. After we digest the initial burst of descriptive and provocative findings, we can look forward to a more critical and strategic approach that uses sleep and dreaming as experiments of nature, as lenses through which to observe consciousness and its vicissitudes on the way to our long awaited rendezvous with brain-mind integration.

The *mediobasal forebrain area,* whose damage by stroke also causes an apparent loss of dreaming, is, like the supramarginal gyrus, one of the regions that imaging studies indicate as selectively active in REM sleep. This region has been considered to be important to motivation through the influences on the frontal forebrain of aminergic systems ascending from the midbrain, and to emotion via its proximity to and interconnection with the limbic system structure in the temporal lobe. Like the supramarginal gyrus, it is as much a crossroads as it is a city, so that damage to it can be expected to cause difficulties of disconnection as much as damage to cell bodies.

Prior to Solms's work, sleep researchers did not suspect this region to be of crucial importance to dreaming even though, as Solms points out, there was evidence in the literature on the effects of deep bifrontal leucotomy, an operation introduced in the 1930s to relieve intractable cases of schizophrenia and severe obsessive-compulsive disorders. According to Solms, a loss of dreaming was sometimes reported, in addition to such side effects as motoric inertia, bland docility, and emotional passivity.

All of these effects, as well as the desired relief of psychosis and aggressiveness, fit together to suggest that dreaming and psychosis are both states characterized by emotion-driven cognition as well as by false perceptions, and raise the possibility that the activation of the emotion and motivational systems of the limbic forebrain have a primary role in shaping the mental content of both abnormal and normal states with these formal features.

In his interpretation of these results, Solms emphasizes the apparent necessity of activating these forebrain emotion and motivation centers as so critical to dreaming that he favors the idea that dreaming occurs if and only if the brain is "motivated." Solms then tries to use this notion to resuscitate Freud's idea that all dreams are wish fulfillments, that the forebrain activation in sleep is caused by dopamine (not acetylcholine), and that the forebrain is capable of creating the conditions necessary for dreaming without the participation of the brain stem. I will examine each of these ideas in turn.

Dreaming as Wish Fulfillments

Freud's original concept was founded on the idea that the unconscious was the dynamically repressed repository of forbidden impulses (the wishes) that were released during sleep. Were it not for their detoxification by disguise and censorship, these alien impulses would awaken the dreamer. This idea has always been difficult to accept because the presence of raw and strongly negative emotion is often *undisguised* in dreams and because the associated dream content is almost always salient to whatever emotion is directing the dream. Furthermore, it is difficult to identify unconscious wishes with motivation in the modern sense of the word. To say that dreaming is motivated, implying activation of the brain circuits for motivation and reward, is not the same as saying that dreaming is driven by unconscious wishes in Freud's intended meaning.

What does seem clear from the new data is that dreaming is driven— strongly—by forebrain systems subserving primary emotions, and that these emotions, are potent shapers of dream plots. The activation of the amygdala, shown by PET studies, is entirely consonant with the phenomenological fact that anxiety is, by far, the leading dream emotion. But anxiety was not a wish for Freud. It was, instead, a symptom caused by conflict about those wishes. In order to retrofit the modern data onto Freud's idea of wish fulfillment as dream instigator, we must inflict considerable damage on the concept of wish fulfillment itself, as well as other aspects of his dream theory and its waking relative, the theory of neurosis. If instead we take the new data to indicate a strong, primary role for the activation of the deep mediobasal substrates of emotion and motivation, the resulting concept fits seamlessly into the activation-synthesis hypothesis.

Now the question is, does the forebrain do any of these things independently of the brain stem?

Motivating the Forebrain and Dopamine

The role of dopamine in the sleep-wake cycle is still, unfortunately, obscure. One hopes Solms will himself take up this important and unresolved issue as a way of testing his intriguing but entirely speculative hypothesis that dreaming can occur if and only if the forebrain dopamine systems are activated. Activation can occur, according to Solms, in any phase of sleep and without the participation of the brain stem caudal to the midbrain sources of dopamine.

The idea that dopamine circuits might be selectively activated in sleep is an intriguing one. Dreaming *is* clearly motivated. Even in the case of its domination by negative affects, dreamers are motivated to *do* something—to flee or to fight, for example. This is not wish fulfillment; sex, the motive that interested Freud the most, is distinctly underrepresented in dreams. Further damaging to Freud's theory is the finding that when sex *is* represented in dreams, it is quite nakedly undisguised, intensely pleasurable, and can even lead to orgasm, whether or not it awakens the dreamer!

As soon as we discovered that both the norepinephrine and serotonin neuromodulatory systems were selectively inactivated in REM sleep, we predicted that this same property might apply to all aminergic systems. It does apply to histamine, but not to dopamine! When we recorded from putative dopamine neurons in the substantia nigra, we were impressed with how little they changed their firing properties in any state! They tended to fire at the same high rates in NREM and REM sleep as they did in waking. We therefore lost interest in them as brain state instigators.

This may have been a premature dismissal, and I hope that Solms's hypothesis will stimulate a new cycle of investigative interest.

What we know so far does not augur well for Solms's hypotheses, however. If dopamine systems are constantly activated, they could supply motivational juice to the brain no matter what state it was in. But other systems would need to be invoked to account for the across-state differences. How could Solms account for the evanescence and intermittency of dreaming, given the apparent constancy of dopamine output? Why, for example, don't we dream as frequently or as intensely in NREM sleep (or in waking, for that matter) if dopamine is playing more than an incidental role in the instigation of dreaming? It could be that dopamine abets the motivational aspects of *both* dreaming and waking cognition. This seems plausible and conforms to the observations in hand.

The other question that the imputation of an active role for dopamine in dreams raises is, where is the dopamine coming from? Although there *are* dopamine cells that innervate local circuits in such forebrain sites as the hypothalamus, all of the dopamine cells which project to the rest of the brain are in the brain stem! What becomes of Solms's theory of the independence of forebrain dream instigators if much or most of the dopamine released there is related to cellular activity in the midbrain?

Whatever the answer to this question, it seems to me reckless to propose that any part of the brain operates independently of any other. This is especially true of a hierarchical system like the reticular thalamic one that controls forebrain activation so prominently. Of course, the several neuronal participants in this hierarchical system will occasionally become dissociated so that now the cortex, now the thalamus, now the brain stem takes the lead in state component generation, but in order for state control to have any reliability, the flow of control *has* to be from the bottom up.

Activation-Synthesis Revisited

The arguments in favor of forebrain mechanisms in dreaming presented here are designed in part to counter the widespread misperception that activation-synthesis regards REM sleep as the exclusive correlate of dreaming, that the forebrain in sleep does only what the brain stem tells it to do, and that dreaming is entirely nonsensical due to the chaotic nature of the brain stem instructions. A careful reading of the original 1977 articulation of the theory and its many subsequent reiterations and revisions will convince any fair-minded reader that all three of these attributions are unwarranted. The original model is shown in figure 9.2.

Let me set the record straight again about what activation-synthesis said then and what AIM now says about these three issues: (1) REM sleep is the state most favorable to dream generation, NREM sleep is intermediate, and waking is the least favorable; (2) the reason for this continuum (which is statistical and quantitative, not absolute and qualitative) is that the strongest determinant of this succession of states is the reciprocal interaction of brainstem aminergic and cholinergic systems; and (3) the changes in cognition that distinguish dreaming from waking—especially the deficits in orientation, directed thought, and memory—derive from the effects of the change in bottom-up inputs that are a product of reciprocal interaction.

The sudden availability of PET imaging and brain lesion data add a welcome and critical new element to the picture, that of differential activation of the forebrain. What is needed now is a concerted effort to appropriately modify our picture of wake-sleep neurophysiology and its relationship to consciousness and its vicissitudes. To make the most of this great opportunity, it is important wherever possible to integrate the new findings with what we know already from basic research in animals and from sleep lab studies in humans. With that goal in mind, I suggest the following integrative hypotheses, some of which are illustrated in figure 9.3.

1. The shift from waking to REM sleep, which is accompanied by changes from alert awareness to dreaming, is occasioned not only by changes in input-output gating and modulation as previously supposed, but also by changes in regional activation of the forebrain.

2. Four changes in regional activation are particularly relevant to understanding the concomitant changes in consciousness:

a. *Selective activation of the supramarginal gyrus in REM sleep* facilitates the intense and convincing visuospatial imagery of our dreams, a distinctive phenomenological feature that has previously gone unexplained except by speculative reference to the PGO waves that selectively activate the posterolateral cortex in cats. The raw visual hallucinatory data, which are processed by the supramarginal gyrus, are generated by the visual associative cortex far downstream from the primary visual cortex. Imaging studies, especially with fMRI techniques, would be useful to explore the possibility that the supramarginal gyrus integrates and/or acts as a way station for the cortical processing of PGO-like phasic activation signals during REM sleep in both humans and animals.

b. *Selective activation of the amygdala in REM sleep* is relevant to the phenomenological fact that dreaming is characterized by strong emotion, principally anxiety (but also elation and anger). The apparently primary activation of the amygdala and adjacent paralimbic cortices further suggests that emotion may be a primary shaper of dream plots, a hypothesis already suggested by the finding that dream cognition, however intrinsically bizarre, is usually consonant with dream emotion. Because we can record PGO activity in both the cholinergic areas of the lateral pons and the amygdala, it is natural to hypothesize that the activation of emotion in dreams is selective because the amygdala is such a prime target of PGO input. Here again, fMRI studies of humans and experimental animals could be quite helpful.

c. *Activation of a wide variety of forebrain structures* including the hypothalamus and medial frontal cortex may potentiate the generation of emotionally salient memories and of important instinctual repertoires in REM sleep. Significantly, the ventromedial prefrontal cortex is the site hypothesized by Antonio Damasio for the matching of emotional and bodily responses to specific events and scenarios that guide our social behavior. Their selective activation could impart to dreaming the virtual enactment of escape, attack, and courtship scenarios of human dreams and allow these psychophysiologic principles to be linked to animal experimental data in a functionally significant way. Animal studies are beginning to look more closely at the hypothalamus and basal forebrain, with some focused questions in mind: Can PGO activity be recorded here in cats? Does dopamine play a special role in REM sleep generation and/or does this region mirror the neuromodulatory profile of the brain stem?

d. *Selective inactivation of the dorsolateral prefrontal cortex* is a capital discovery that was completely unanticipated by basic sleep research. This data helps our effort to understand the bizarreness, the loss of volition, the loss of self-reflection, the loss of directed thought, and the amnesia of dreaming that we have previously attributed to the shift in neuromodulatory balance of the brain. Now we can entertain the strong and attractively reductive hypothesis that these two mechanisms are both synergistic and mechanistically integral. In retrospect, perhaps we should have made more of the fact that the frontal cortex is the only area of the forebrain that appears *not* to be invaded by PGO waves.

When we take PGO waves to be evidence of cholinergically mediated phasic activation, we can suggest that the frontal cortex is the one area of the cat brain that is selectively deprived of this distinctive REM sleep activation process. Here again, a comparative study, using f MRI imaging, might yield surprisingly consonant results.

The central hypothesis linking all four of these integrative propositions is that the regional activation differences may well reflect the differential targeting of the forebrain region by *both* phasic activation waves (PGO equivalents) and by differential distribution of cholinergic and monoaminergic inputs to the forebrain. The combined effects of these two processes could include selective neuronal activation and inactivation, direct and indirect redirection of local blood flow, and regional differences in intracellular chemical events mediated by differential second messenger influences.

Temporal Lobe Epilepsy (TLE)

The fact that the temporal lobe is selectively activated in REM sleep in humans and is the target of phasic activation waves in REM sleep in animals begs comparison to the classic description of the states that may suddenly interrupt waking consciousness in patients with temporal lobe epilepsy. Temporal lobe epilepsy is caused by the phasic discharge of intrinsic neuronal circuits whose excitability has been altered, usually owing to damage to neighboring neurons—presumably those normally exerting an inhibitory influence on their epileptic progenitors.

The general hypothesis that we now wish to consider is that this disease process (which is the reciprocal of stroke damage) causes the temporal lobe more readily to enter a condition of phasic excitability increase akin to that which normally occurs only in REM sleep. If losses of dreaming occur with stroke damage to this region, does a corresponding increase in the intensity of dreaming occur in patients with temporal epilepsy? The answer, according to Mark Solms, appears to be yes. A related question, to which the answer must remain speculative, is whether the dreamy states of temporal lobe patients are the consequences of a physiological process homologous to REM sleep that occurs in waking. What are the reasons for taking these two questions seriously?

The PGO waves of REM sleep are epileptiform. Both consist of spike and wave EEG complexes that are morphologically indistinguishable. In both PGO waves and temporal lobe epilepsy, these spike and wave complexes are generated by similar mechanisms: owing to a physiological decline in inhibitory modulation (REM sleep) or to structural damage (TLE), neurons are disinhibited and fire in intense bursts, of which the EEG spike and wave complex is the extracellular record.

Common mechanisms appear to link the two similar EEG phenomena. In the case of REM sleep, the disinhibition is due, in part, to the noradrenergic and serotonergic neuronal firing arrest and to the consequent increase in excitability of neurons, including cholinergic ones. It is quite likely that these changes are related also to shifts in GABAergic inhibition and glutaminergic excitation, as is the case in temporal lobe epilepsy. From an experimental point of view, an effective way to kindle epilepsy is to weaken the aminergic modulatory inputs to the temporal lobe, and some have even suggested that inducing permanent changes in neuromodulatory balance in the temporal lobe produces kindling.

As to the phenomenology, normal dreams and the pathological dreamy states of epilepsy share the following formal features:

1. There is a loss of contact with the outside world and a retreat into the virtual reality of the dream(y) state.

2. Hallucinations are quite common and often consist of vivid and sharply detailed visual imagery in both dreams and seizure states.

3. Bizarre cognition occurs frequently in both conditions and is characterized by discontinuities, and incongruities of imagined times, places, and people.

4. One may experience strong emotion, especially fear, elation, and anger.

5. The subjective experiences are evanescent and difficult to recall at their termination.

Arthur Epstein has emphasized and described this formal analogy, with many colorfully detailed examples, in his book entitled *Dreaming and Other Involuntary Mentation*. For neuropsychiatrist Epstein, the analogy is strongly supportive of such psychoanalytic constructs as the release of libidinal impulses, primary process thinking, and dreaming as the symbolic manifestation of the same. For the cognitive neuroscientist, the analogy serves simply to bring two apparently diverse phenomena into the same brain-mind state space. These viewpoints are not mutually exclusive, especially if we keep in mind Freud's early injunctions to honor the brain.

As Mark Solms points out in his recent book, the dreams of patients with temporal lobe epilepsy *are* more intense than those of normals. They are more frequently intensely unpleasant or nightmarish, and this is presumably a function of higher levels of anxiety mediated by the hyperexcitable amygdala of the epileptic patients. These hypotheses are testable in two ways. One is to confirm the anecdotal reports of patients by studying the subjects in sleep labs, as José Calvo and his group have done in Mexico City. Compared to age- and sex-matched controls, the epileptic subjects had measurably higher levels of anxiety in their dream reports.

The other way to test the interaction between seizure propensity and dream intensity is to perform brain imaging experiments in temporal lobe patients, as Lia Silvestri and our group have begun to do in Boston. By injecting a radioisotope when the patient is in REM sleep and comparing the resulting SPECT image to that obtained during resting and waking, we can quantify the activation levels of the temporal lobes in both states and compare them to one another. Our results are still very preliminary, but they suggest that the temporal lobe that carries the epileptic focus is even more highly activated in REM than the nonepileptic lobe, as if the epileptic propensity in the already disinhibited, diseased lobe potentiated the normal REM sleep drive toward paroxysmal discharge.

Temporal lobe epilepsy thus represents a cruel experiment of nature whose study, using the tools and concepts of modern sleep science, may yield valuable insights. For example, it seems quite possible that by pushing the temporal lobe toward the more paroxysmal discharge mode, REM sleep constitutes a provocative test of seizure vulnerability that could substitute for the more difficult diagnostic test of recording a spontaneous seizure in waking. As a corollary, we could quantify response to medication using the REM sleep intensification measure as a bioassay. Other important clinical questions involve the effects of seizures and abnormal REM sleep on sleep dependent effects on cognition. Because the temporal lobe and adjacent subcortical structures appear to be crucial to the organization and maintenance of emotionally salient memories, it would not be surprising to find that long-term seizure processes caused progressive dysfunction in this domain.

Alcohol, Sleep, and Delirium Tremens

Even normal people can be pushed to the limit of seizures through the abuse of drugs or alcohol. In these cases the seizures usually develop in the period of withdrawal, suggesting that they reflect alterations in the excitability of the brain that have taken place during the period of abuse but that are not expressed until the chemical that actually causes them is taken away. In order to maintain the desired alteration in consciousness afforded by the drug *and* to suppress the unpleasant effects of withdrawal, addicts typically increase their intake until the time of crisis inevitably occurs. It thus seems quite likely that the drug effectively quells the seizures that the withdrawal syndrome induces.

As we will see in part V, the Recreational Drugstore, many of the abused stimulant drugs that cause seizures during acute use are highly sleep suppressant through their direct action on neuromodulatory systems. Alcohol, by contrast, is a general central nervous system suppressant. As such, and in contrast to the stimulants, alcohol causes euphoria only as a relatively brief consequence of its essentially anesthetic action on the brain. By numbing the brain it induces relaxation, lifts cortical inhibition, and produces a temporary sense of comfort with the self and with society.

One consequence of the CNS suppressant effect of alcohol is sedation. Alcohol is sedative through its facilitation of NREM sleep physiology, namely EEG spindles and slow waves. This is what makes alcohol so popular among insomniacs. But alcohol is a very poor sedative for two complementary reasons: it suppresses REM sleep, and its breakdown products (which peak two to three hours post ingestion) are highly arousing, causing the early morning awakenings that are often the first definite sign of hangover. It seems quite likely that the brain is, already, going down the slippery slope toward seizures and delirium tremens.

This process is readily reversed by abstinence. Following an acute overdose of alcohol, recovery sleep is often deep, refreshing, and full of dreams. This rebound effect is typical of any intervention that temporarily impedes REM. The physiological payback is prompt and precise. But the process is perpetuated—and aggravated—by repeated alcohol use. "Hair of the dog" is the quasi-homeopathic slogan tied to drinking that fateful "eye-opener" the morning after. The fact that the noxious feelings of hangover—controlled by a second dose of alcohol—would normally give way to sleepiness, a nap, and REM rebound, renders more plausible the hypothesis that REM suppression is an integral and not just an incidental part of the addiction-withdrawal cycle.

In any case, it is quite clear that REM suppression is a robust consequence of prolonged alcohol abuse. This effect becomes increasingly problematic as the addiction is prolonged and the inevitable crisis is made worse even as it is postponed. Barbiturates, another CNS depressant sedative class of drug, offer a similar picture. When barbiturates are used experimentally to suppress REM—and they are *very* effective REM suppressants—their dose frequency and amount must be increased more and more over time until, at 3–4 weeks, it is virtually impossible to quell the REM rebound. When it finally occurs, it is characterized by such intense phasic activation (PGO waves) that the animals literally fly off their sleeping surfaces in convulsive spasms.

Humans who hit the wall of alcohol withdrawal show the more complex picture of toxic-delirium, consisting of visual hallucinations (often with stereotyped insect and animal imagery like the bugs and pink elephants of barfly lore), disorientation and confusion, confabulation, and memory loss as their seizure propensity increases.

Sleep lab recordings reveal that in the first three days following alcohol withdrawal, the REM sleep rebound becomes so intense as to practically displace the NREM sleep that alcohol had initially enhanced at the expense of REM. This is REM debt payback with a vengeance. As the subject becomes more and more tremulous, more and more delirious, and more and more seizure prone, REM sleep levels go to 100 percent of sleep, indicating a marked shift in brain excitability that we assume is related to a desperate attempt of the system to restore neuromodulatory equilibrium.

Whether we should see the ultimate breakthrough of psychosis as the eruption of REM processes into waking or as a waking state driven into the REM domain of the state space is unclear. But there is one aspect of delirium tremens that we need to highlight in the context of this formulation, and that is the loss of thermal equilibrium that is often so severe as to be life threatening in delirium tremens sufferers. At crisis, and especially in the summer time, body temperature may suddenly shoot up to

105 or even 106 degrees, threatening literally to cook the brain (hippocampus neurons die at 108!).

We don't know the basis of this loss of temperature control, but we do know that REM sleep is itself associated with failure of the central thermostat, and we know that REM sleep deprivation also causes a loss of temperature. A unifying hypothesis is that any condition that potentiates REM sleep physiology may also compromise the central regulation of body temperature. Relevant to this hypothesis is the fact that the two brain stem aminergic neuromodulators that are inactivated in REM sleep are active in responding to thermal stress.

Because this same psychotic picture—or parts of it—can become a permanent state of consciousness in former alcohol abusers, it seems quite possible that the acute effects push the brain into a part of the state space from which it cannot escape if it has gone there too often or stays there too long. This may be still another warning that the long-term use of any chemical that alters consciousness through effects on brain neuromodulatory systems can incur pathological changes that are at first only functional but later become structural. In the case of alcohol, it is clear that the structural damage, functional impairment and eventual recovery all involve mesolimbic reward circuits linking the midbrain and the limbic system, raising our suspicions that we are being shown a final common path that unites dreaming and delirium, or at least situates them in a common state space whose parameters are defined by activation (including the regional differentiation thereof), input-output stimulus gating (with special emphasis on the tendency to generate potent and preemptive internal stimuli), and modulation (including dopamine in the well-known aminergic and cholinergic sleep-wake system).

The three kinds of disease process we have surveyed in this chapter are the natural analogues of experimental probes of the brain systems that normally alter brain states in animals. Not surprisingly, they alter consciousness in informative ways in humans. Strokes are the equivalent of electrolytic and excitatory neurotoxic lesions; seizures are the equivalent of direct electrical and chemical stimulation; alcohol is the equivalent of parenteral drug administration. In reading across the three disease classes in search of unifying concepts, I hope to stimulate a new era of experimental work in animals, as well as to celebrate what we have accomplished in the arena of human neuropsychology.

One golden opportunity that beckons to us is to create an animal model (or models) for the exploitation of brain imaging methods in the study of conscious state alteration. A first question to ask is: Do the homologues of the brain regions that are selectively activated—and inactivated in man—show the same patterns in animals? Given the stereotyped consistency of sleep cycle neurophysiology across all mammalian species, it would be surprising if the answer were not affirmative. But whatever the answer, developing an imaging probe would enable us to correlate the known patterns of selective cellular and EEG activation and inactivation with the blood flow data. This strategy would serve to calibrate the imaging probe and allow it to be mapped onto the cellular as well as the regional level of analysis. At this time, this connection is nonexistent or, at best, very weak.

Of the existing imaging approaches, the most promising in terms of both temporal and spatial resolution is functional MRI. Powerful 4 tesla magnets are now being used in vision research to identify in man the equivalent of ocular dominance columns whose existence was first established in animals. Success in this venture encourages its application to the study of REM sleep visual system activation in humans and in animals. A good focal point for this work could be the search in both cats and humans for the fMRI-level equivalent of the phasic activation PGO waves so prominent in the REM sleep of cats. Their discovery—which seems almost inevitable, despite the failure to identify them definitively using even very sophisticated EEG methods—would provide the necessary bridge between the cellular and regional levels of analysis.

Part IV
The Medical Drugstore

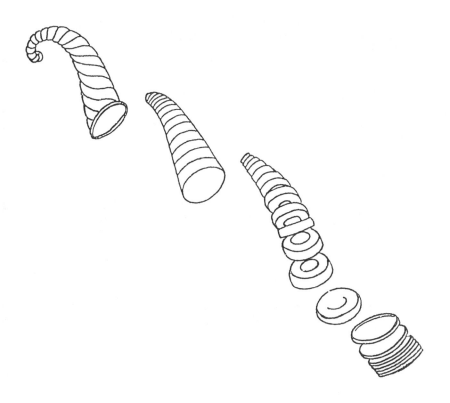

10

The Psychopharmacology of Everyday Life: Drugs for Anxiety and Sleep

The easiest brain-mind principle of all to grasp is this fundamental rule of psychopharmacology: many of the drugs currently prescribed by psychiatrists and other physicians treating patients for psychiatric problems act on the brain-mind state control systems of the brain stem. What this means is that the most potent legal drugs in use today share common mechanisms with the illegal ones. A corollary of this principle is that the differences between legal and illegal drugs are never as sharp as the authorities who make and enforce the laws would have us believe.

But it is not so much my point here to open a political debate about drug use and abuse as it is to define and develop the scientific principles that are at the root of that debate: if you want to alter consciousness, whether it be for fun, for mischief, or for a patient's benefit, you choose a molecule that interacts directly or indirectly with the neuromodulatory systems involved in the spontaneous and innate alterations of consciousness that we all experience as we cycle through waking, sleeping, and dreaming every day and night of our lives.

In this chapter we will see that this Dream Drugstore concept powerfully unites basic neurobiology with clinical psychopharmacology and recreational drug use through the brain-mind state paradigm. Before demonstrating the power of this concept by considering the major disorders of the brain-mind and the various classes of drug that are used to treat them, it is important to highlight several points that cut across all of them. We can conveniently group these ponts in three clusters.

Spatial Considerations Affecting Localization of Drug Action

A shared problem of the street-drug taker and the pill doctor's patient is difficulty delivering the chemical agent to the desired target site in the brain. The problem is that when taken by mouth—or even shot up intravenously—the drugs go everywhere in the body, and that means everywhere in the brain. This is the main reason for the frequency of side effects in the drugs.

Nature is economical in her means. She uses many of the same chemicals to accomplish her nervous purposes within the brain that she has already used to the same ends throughout the body. The good news is that once you have worked out the biochemistry and pharmacology of a neuromodulator in the body, you can apply a lot of what you know to its action in the brain. The bad news is that every time you target, for example, the acetylcholine system of the brain, you also hit the body. That means that the heart, the bowel, the salivary glands, and all the rest of the organs innervated by the autonomic nervous system are influenced. What is worse, the target sites within the brain may not only be as spatially dispersed as in the periphery, but may also be as functionally differentiated!

The REM sleep modulator, acetylcholine, serves to illustrate this issue: in one part of the brain stem (the pons) it promotes sleep; in others (the midbrain and medulla) it promotes waking. This may help explain an apparent paradox: that blocking endogenous acetylcholine with a drug like atropine can induce delirium in waking, whereas endogenous acetylcholine actively mediates the delirium of dreaming! To add richness to this mix, recall that the synthetic cholinergic agonist carbachol greatly enhances REM sleep when injected into highly localized brainstem sites but suppresses it in others and that all of these effects are blocked by atropine. The chemical structure of these molecules is shown in figure 10.1.

How can enhancement and blockade of the same system result in such dissimilar alterations in consciousness? In the case of acetylcholine, we find the answer not only in spatial differentiation, but also in the fact that acetylcholine activates the cortex in both waking and REM sleep but has quite different effects on consciousness because of the other neuromodulators serotonin and norepinephrine that are (in waking) or are not (in REM sleep) co-released.

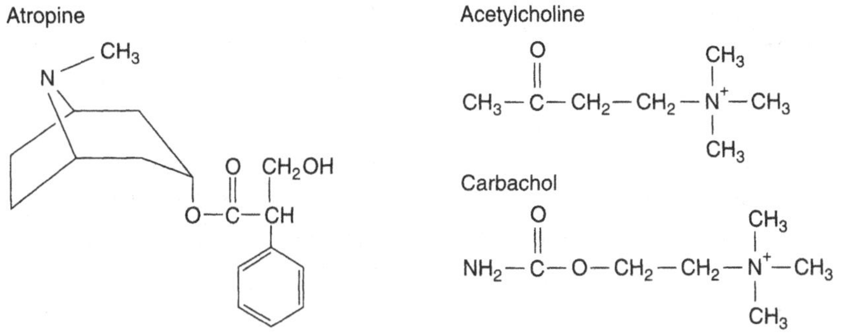

Atropine

Acetylcholine

Figure 10.1
Acetylcholine, carbachol, and atropine. Naturally occurring acetylcholine and its synthetic agonists (e.g., carbachol) and antagonists (e.g., atropine) all share a methylated nitrogen atom which occupies receptor sites so as to mimic (carbachol) or block (atropine) the action of acetylcholine.

The main point of this discussion is that clinical pharmacology as we practice it today is much less spatially precise than the basic science neuropharmacology that informs our model building in the brain-mind state paradigm. This means both that we have a long way to go before we achieve a perfect fit between our mechanistic hypotheses and our clinical observations, and that clinical experiments are not always good ways to test basic science theories.

Considerations Affecting Timing of Drug Administration and of Drug Action

The brain changes its mind continuously. Because we live on the surface of a whirling planet, we experience constantly changing levels of light and temperature with a peak and a trough, each occurring about once every 24 hours as our place on earth comes in and out of opposition to the sun. To adapt to this cosmic rhythm, all living things have evolved an internal rhythm that guarantees a strategic synchronization of their rest and activity with the availability of external energy.

Because the internal rhythm has a period of about 24 hours, it is called *circadian* (meaning about one day in duration). In higher animals, including humans, this circadian rest-activity rhythm is controlled by a specialized part of the hypothalamus in the upper brain stem called the suprachiasmatic nucleus. It has this name because it sits above the cross-ing point of the two optic nerves that carry visual data to the brain, in-cluding the signal that resets the internal rhythm each day as the length of the light period changes.

Waking consciousness is normally associated with the activity phase of the circadian rhythm; sleeping and dreaming consciousness are associated with the rest phase. This coordination is effected by linking the circadian clock in the hypothalamus to the NREM-REM sleep cycle control system in the lower brain stem. Because the linkage is made in part via the major neuromodulatory systems, our propensity to alterations in conscious state varies in a circadian manner and is more or less susceptible to one sort of drug or another, depending upon the circadian phase of the neuro-modulatory system that is its target. All of the major neuromodulatory players in conscious state control vary in a circadian manner.

To understand this principle, consider two examples: (1) the natural time-window for sleep readiness, and (2) the natural time-window for hallucinatory activity. These are important to recognize if we wish either to promote sleep and/or to reduce hallucinosis. Some people sup-pose that they can fall asleep at any time, others that they can fall asleep only at one particular time. Both groups are wrong. Despite wide individ-ual variation in sleep proneness—as measured by the multiple sleep la-tency test—there are both windows of opportunity (the mid to late afternoon) and forbidden zones (the mid evening) for sleep that affect all of us. I am sleepy now at 4:15 P.M., but four hours from now (at 8:15 P.M.), I won't be sleepy at all! Both of these probabilities depend upon the circadian curves of body temperature. The way in which the circadian rhythm may interact with AIM so as to produce these effects is shown in figure 10.2.

Like sleep, hallucinatory propensity also fluctuates, reaching its peak in the early morning hours when the circadian propensity for REM sleep is nearing its zenith. One might think that the peak of REM propensity would occur during sleep, but it doesn't. If subjects can fall asleep at all, the tendency for that sleep to be REM continues to rise until 11:00 A.M., well after the normal time of awakening. So one problem that all drug users face is their own constantly altered physiological propensity to be in one state of consciousness or another. A corollary problem is that the drugs they take are present in their blood for widely ranging time periods.

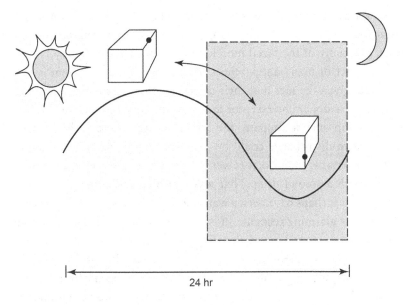

Figure 10.2
Circadian process and AIM. The circadian (~24 hr) curve of body temperature is shown in its entrained mode to illustrate the combined effects of light and temperature on AIM. At the zenith of the temperature curve waking is favored while following the nadir, REM sleep is favored.

The Half-Life of Drugs

Drugs that alter conscious states have varying time courses of action that are usually measured as "half-lives," defined as the time it takes for the blood level of the drug to fall to 50 percent of its peak level. Sedatives are classed as short-, medium-, and long-acting according to their half-lives of about 2, 4, and 6 hours. A complicating factor is the second wave of effects, usually undesirable, that may follow as the drug is metabolized. As with alcohol, this second wave of metabolite-induced effects can be both psychonoxious and hangover-like. The price paid for prolonged sedation may be malaise and poor performance the following day.

But the most insidious effects are in the third wave of long-delayed changes of the sort that we see with the antipsychotic drugs that have been taken for long periods of time. These changes often affect the motor system and may even outlast discontinuation of the drug. The best known of these is called tardive dyskinesia (delayed movement disorder). Tardive dyskinesia was first observed in the 1970s, when the phenothiazines had been in use for 10–15 years. The syndrome consists of involuntary movements, especially of the facial muscles, and Parkinsonian rigidity.

The impact of many antipsychotic drugs on the motor system is not surprising, given the fact that their desirable effects are directly proportional to their dopamine receptor antagonism. Sometimes acute Parkinson-like symptoms accompany the initial dosing. Those early signs of motor system disturbance could be countered by giving anticholinergic agents like Artane. Thus doctors were treating a drug-induced functional disorder with a second drug. That was alarming enough and, in retrospect, should perhaps have been a warning signal of worse things to come.

An equally alarming recognition is now growing in the case of the far more widely prescribed mood-elevating drugs, the selective serotonin reuptake blockers (or SSRIs). These drugs are used to alleviate depression, obsessive compulsive disorder, or even as "cosmetic" agents for the competitive urbanite seeking an energy boost. As with tardive dyskinesia, there is a two-phase scenario. In phase I, the eye movements of sleep are affected. Instead of being restricted to the REM periods, they occur throughout sleep, resulting in severe disorganization of sleep architecture. Because the only symptomatic effect of the Phase I sleep motor disturbance is a sense of continuous dreaming, patients usually accept it in exchange for the daytime high that goes with it. So far so good. Or, at least, so far not so bad.

But later, in Phase II, after two years of continuous use, the SSRIs may contribute to a more ominous motor syndrome, the REM sleep behavior disorder described in chapter 8 as the enactment of dreamed movement. For reasons still not well understood, the drugs interfere with our normal ability to inhibit motor outputs. As with tardive dyskinesia victims, patients who develop SSRI-induced RBD may find that their sleep disorder does not abate when they discontinue the drug. The RBD can itself be treated with benzodiazepines—Clonazepam, for example. But that may be throwing good drug money after bad. And a more disturbing possibility, not yet observed, is that the SSRI-induced RBD will evolve in the same way that spontaneous RBD does: to full-blown Parkinson's disease.

It is too early to know if such alterations in consciousness—the tendency to enact dreaming in RBD—are permanent. Forever, as the song points out, is a long, long time! But the handwriting is on the wall, and it reads as follows.

The neuromodulatory systems of the brain stem directly alter normal states of consciousness such that we experience psychosis-like phenomena in our dreams. Drugs that increase or decrease the efficacy of any one of these systems are therefore likely to be quite effective in achieving desirable shifts in the cognitive and emotional symptoms of spontaneous alterations of consciousness like schizophrenia and depression. These benefits may come at a price, however, because other state components are always tied to cognition and emotion at a deep mechanistic level. Long-term use of neuromodulatory agonists or antagonists may reset the system in compensatory modes that are very difficult to reverse.

The sad conclusion is that the medical profession and the pharmaceutical industry may be collaborating in an unwitting and unplanned program of experimental medicine. For those physician-scientists at the interface of neurology and psychiatry who are interested in consciousness, the opportunities presented for understanding are strongly countered by the ethical dilemmas raised. Is it reasonable to expect that tampering with neuromodulation in such a crude way will ever be without risk? How many cases of long-lasting side effects need to be observed before a more urgent alarm is sounded? What now constitutes fully informed consent in putting normal subjects into studies of these drugs?

It is ironic, to say the least, to note that some of those concerns raised about the psychedelic drugs that led to their being made illegal now apply equally strongly to entirely legal therapeutic agents. One inescapable conclusion is that the line between legality and illegality is so fine in this case as to vanish. Does that mean that in the interests of consistency we should make all the drugs legal? Or should they all be made illegal? The political, social, and ethical implications of these questions are mind-boggling. To develop an informed approach, we need to look more closely at some aspects of clinical pharmacology.

Clean and Dirty Drugs

For scientific reasons, it is always desirable to focus on one and only one thing in any given experiment. In psychopharmacology, this desideratum is expressed in so-called "clean" drugs that have one and only one action.

"Dirty" drugs are those that affect more than one brain system. But it should already be apparent that simply on the grounds of reciprocal interaction there is no such thing as a clean drug once the pill has been swallowed. This is because even the pharmacological purity earned by a drug's selectivity for a given neuromodulator or a single receptor is immediately sullied by the complex dynamics of neurophysiology. Change the acetylcholine system and you immediately change the dopamine, serotonin, and norepinephrine systems. This could be varied at least three ways by substituting any one of the aminergic modulators for acetylcholine: each of them interacts dynamically with those of all the others.

To facilitate the interpretation of pharmacological data it is useful to know that a drug acts in a highly specific way. We can see specificity at several levels: the drug must be able to pass the blood-brain barrier; once in the brain, the drug should interact with only one neuromodulatory system; and, best of all, it should bind to one and only one receptor subtype. Basic pharmacology has every reason to seek such specificity in the design of drugs and to applaud its discovery when it is found.

Extension of this specificity principle to the clinical domain has resulted in the availability of increasingly well-aimed chemical bullets. If we wanted to block just one of the many serotonin receptors to see what would happen, we could probably do it! But if we wanted to elevate mood in depression—or obsessive-compulsive disorder—would we expect the best result if we blocked just that one receptor? And if we wanted to discourage auditory hallucinations in schizophrenia, would we want our drug to target only D2 dopamine receptors, even if we knew that the antipsychotic action of drugs correlated well with a drug's affinity for those receptors?

In other words, does pharmacological purity always predict clinical efficacy? It certainly would if the mind or any one of its many altered states were mediated by a single species of neuromodulator or a single receptor. That medical scientists might think so is understandable, given the strength and success of the one-gene one-enzyme model of diseases like phenylketonuria. But the mind and its many altered states are not only not known to be so mediated, but they are known *not* to be so mediated. Take dreaming as a case in point. It requires the harmonious and often contrapuntal orchestration of at least three of the four major neuromodulatory systems to turn on and off.

The upshot is that a better drug for increasing dreaming or decreasing psychosis might be one that simultaneously and directly played on two, three, or even more neuromodulatory systems simultaneously. That means that a better drug might be a dirtier one! This is not an endorsement of carelessness nor is it to suggest that knowing whether a drug is clean or dirty is not important. It is, rather, a turning of the reductionistic model on its head by saying that because the mind and its states are emergent properties of complex systems, it follows that we may need to design the most effective pharmacological interventions to play on more than one system in more than one way! This is indeed the case in some antidepressants and in the novel antipsychotics.

Perhaps the best example of this principle is the new antipsychotic drug, clozaril, which works on the serotonin and norepinephrine, as well as on the dopamine systems. Clozaril is a *very* dirty drug, and yet patients with severe schizophrenic psychoses—unresponsive to any of the cleaner neuroleptics—have been effectively treated with it. Once you have seen a patient who has been socially withdrawn and severely delusional for years suddenly conversing normally you quickly abandon the canon of pharmacological purity.

A corollary of this point is that the brain itself is not only dirty (in that it consists of multiple, often competing systems wired up in parallel), but that it is *also* dirty (via the serial principle of adaptation). Effects at time A almost certainly lead to opposite or quite different effects at time B, and so on. This means that when we give a drug we change the system by setting in motion a sequence of effects whose endpoints are quite unpredictable (if indeed there are any endpoints!). In this case, "dirty" is not a good thing if either the unpredictable effects are undesirable or irreversible or—heaven forbid—both. But just this double trouble appears to plague patients with tardive dyskinesia, the example already discussed in terms of temporal factors.

With all of these caveats in mind, the reader may well wonder who has the heart or the stomach to dispense or to take drugs that, however legally, alter consciousness in such wild and uncontrolled ways. I have already confessed to my own cowardliness as drug taker and drug prescriber. You have to make up your own mind about where you stand on these issues. All that I hope to do now is share some observations and thoughts about how some of the most widely used drugs may alter consciousness in ways that are interesting, useful, and sometimes problematical.

The Benzodiazepines

In the 1970s, three of the top ten best-selling drugs in the United States were Librium, Valium, and Dalmane. All were benzodiazepines manufactured by Roche Laboratories. The result of a serendipitous discovery by Roche chemist Leo Sternbach, these drugs are of scientific importance because they demonstrate that an exogenous chemical can enhance the dissociation between anxiety and arousal normally seen in sleep and waking. At first glance, this pill option looked far better than relaxation, meditation, or psychotherapy, because it allowed the user to continue to lead a stress-filled life without being slowed down by the nagging signal of anxiety. At about twice the anxiolytic dose, the benzodiazepines were also effective sedatives, and some of them were successfully marketed as such, often to the same fast-lane users that used them as "tranquilizers" in the daytime. What a bonanza for the marketing folk: take one pill to quiet the jangle of frayed nerves in the daytime, and two more to stop the noise at night.

Sternbach opened the benzodiazepine revolution when he observed that chlordiazepoxide (Librium) was a potent anti-anxiety agent despite the fact that the process used in its synthesis had changed it from the quinazoline class that Sternbach had wanted to study into a completely new kind of molecule. The investigation of the benzodiazepines has since revealed the surprising presence in the brain of receptors for the drugs in the same chloride ion channel protein that mediates many drugs' sedative and anticonvulsant effects. It is significant for our story that the highest concentration of benzodiazepine receptors is in the limbic system, particularly the amygdala.

Uncoupling Arousal and Anxiety

The recent history of psychopharmacology has been driven by the quest for drugs that could relieve anxiety without producing sedation. Not surprisingly, anxiety and arousal normally go hand in hand. Because anxiety is an internally generated alarm signal, it generally leads to an alerting response. This is adaptive. It tells the organism to stop, look, and listen

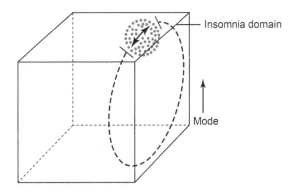

Figure 10.3
Anxiety and insomnia. Anxiety opposes entry into sleep because the aminergic drive is kept elevated and subjects are frozen at the wake-sleep interface.

in order to detect the cause for alarm, identify it, and reduce or eliminate it. But many an anxious person may not be able to detect the cause for alarm, and some may not even want to do so. Hence the popularity of the benzodiazepines.

Which is cause and which is effect? In some models, the arousal is secondary to the anxiety. But if the subject ignores or can't reduce the anxiety signal and overrides it and so maintains high levels of arousal, anxiety persists and may even augment, suggesting that there is positive feedback in both directions. This normally tight linkage between arousal and anxiety has led many neuroscientists to suppose that the brain stem systems mediating arousal might co-mediate the anxiety. In particular, some hold that the locus coeruleus, in response to arousing stimuli from within or without, activates the limbic system (triggering anxiety) in parallel with the thalamocortical system (triggering arousal). The dynamics of this process are illustrated in figure 10.3.

But the fact that we experience anxiety—often of panic proportions in our REM sleep dreams when the locus coeruleus is shut down completely—means two things: that arousal—at least in the waking sense of the term—and anxiety are completely dissociable; and that the brain-mind is capable of generating anxiety without the help of the locus coeruleus! In fact, REM sleep dream anxiety cannot depend upon norepinephrine, or serotonin, or histamine either, which leaves dopamine and acetylcholine as the only two neuromodulatory candidates for anxiety mediation. The fact that both are active in waking and REM, the two states in which we experience anxiety, is consistent with a mediating role, but of course does not prove it. Besides uncoupling anxiety and arousal when taken at low doses during waking, the benzodiazepines turned out to be able to induce sedation if they were taken at higher doses at bedtime.

One reason for Roche's success with Dalmane was that it did not share two undesirable features of the barbiturates, the then reigning class of sedatives: REM suppression and suicidal potency. The barbiturates are CNS depressants that can induce unconsciousness, but because they have a very low margin of safety they can also shut down the respiratory control system of the brain stem. That is how they kill, and that is why they are still popular in Oregon and other places where individuals are free to elect a definitive end to unbearably unpleasant conscious awareness. Physician-assisted suicide is sometimes accomplished by turning off breathing, by pulling the plug internally as it were.

Many scientists do not recognize that because the respiratory system is a specialized subdivision of the brain stem activating system, its functioning is intrinsically state dependent. This drive to breathe rises and falls with levels of brain stem activation and arousal, and the level of arousal rises and falls with the level of respiration. Maybe that's why the voluntary control of respiration is so key in altering consciousness. When bidding for calm and patient reflection, we say "take a deep breath," and we intentionally lower our breathing rate when seeking the tranquillity of the relaxation response. In any case, the benzodiazepines do not exert their sedative effects by knocking out the brain stem activating system. Even when they produce coma they may not impede respiration. That is why they have such a low suicidal potential.

Barbiturates were also undesirable because, even at relatively low sedative doses, they suppressed REM sleep. As with that popular CNS depressant alcohol, whenever REM is actively suppressed, a debt is incurred. The increased REM pressure induced by deprivation inevitably leads either to violent rebound (if the drug is stopped) or to the breakthrough of dreamlike mentation into waking as the pressure becomes irrepressible. When the disorganizing effects of REM sleep dream breakthrough finally make drug seeking behavior impossible, a psychotic delirium, along with the seizures famously known as "rum fits" may be precipitated. The benzodiazepines were thus touted as safer (true), more physiological (questionable) sedatives because they did not suppress REM in normal subjects even though they can be used to control dream enactment in the REM sleep behavior disorder.

Now it is probably no coincidence that in addition to occupying the benzodiazepine receptor site on the chloride ion channel protein, these remarkable drugs can also occupy the sedation-convulsant receptor of the same protein. Sedation with benzodiazepines thus goes hand in hand with anticonvulsant power—as if the two processes had some deep mediating mechanism in common with each other. What could that be?

One obvious answer is the tendency to synchronization of neuronal circuits that is characteristic of both NREM sleep and generalized seizures. The term synchronization refers to the widespread and concerted rhythmic firing that takes the brain-mind out of contact with the world at sleep and seizure onset. That synchronization may well be a common mechanism is supported by the observation—not promulgated by the drug companies—the benzodiazepines suppress stages III and IV of NREM sleep, even if they do not suppress REM. Stages III and IV are the most highly synchronized phases of sleep and the most comalike. On benzodiazepines we may fall asleep earlier and stay asleep longer, but we sleep less deeply.

So the benzodiazepines produce unphysiological sleep. Do they knock out growth and sex hormone release along with stages III and IV? We don't know the answers to these questions, but if I were pubescent I would assume they might and think about the possible consequences.

Even at my advanced age, I would be cautious about the benzodiazepines, because they have two other problematic features: rebound insomnia and drug dependency. These two related defects make it hard to stop using the benzodiazepines because your sleep is sometimes worse when you try to stop than it was before you started. That is a strong inducement to resume drug taking, especially if the insomnia is coupled with daytime anxiety, fatigue, and poor concentration. That's why I always urge my patients to get good and tired in some sleep promoting way, like jogging, biking, or making love, before they commit themselves to a pill. Such activities are naturally sleep enhancing as well as entertaining.

Another intriguing link between sleep and anxiety lies in the distribution of benzodiazepine receptors in the brain. Given their selective anxiolytic power—at first sparing sleep—where would you expect them to be heavily concentrated? In the limbic lobe, of course. And that's exactly where they are! Not in the brain stem, and not in the cortex. In limbic structures—and in the amygdala at that! The amygdala, you will recall, is a limbic structure that is selectively activated in REM, a finding that helps us explain the surges of anxiety in REM sleep dreams!

If the benzodiazepines shift the amygdala-dorsolateral prefrontal cortex balance in favor of the cortex during waking, we could easily understand why anxiety is quelled while executive cognitive functions are preserved (when people take them in low doses). They make waking more wake-like and less dreamlike. Thus they might confer a two-pronged competitive advantage on the overachiever's consciousness: enhancing concentration and suppressing worry. But remember, there is no free lunch in the Dream Drugstore. In exchange for tuning out anxiety by day and turning out your lights by night, you might distort your sleep and you might get hooked by these magical molecules.

Frank Berger, one of the scientists who discovered the first anxiolytic drug, was horrified that so many people sought to solve what he considered to be problems in living by popping pills. Of his own drug discovery, meprobamate, he said:

They are widely prescribed merely to ease problems of living. They may be effective for this purpose [only] to the extent that they dull sensibility to the knocks, annoyances and frustrations of everyday life. When used in this manner they are being used . . . not as antianxiety drugs. I find it difficult to believe that the self-confidence needed to cope with one's problems can be acquired by the use of any medication. (p. 291 in Berger, 1981)

But of course the drug companies laughed all the way to the bank!

11

Regulating Mood: The MAOIs, Tricyclics, and SSRIs

In developing the brain-mind state paradigm, I have repeatedly empha-sized the tight link between emotion and cognition. Nowhere is that link more clear than in the influence that mood or feeling state has upon think-ing. Depression drains the brain of energy, and when it does so, it both slows thought processes and subverts them to the blackest and most dire preoccupations. Even those of us who have never experienced clinical depression know that our minds can be changed—for the worse—by dis-couraging news, by the loss of love and loved ones, and even by the loss of sun in winter.

It is as if our consciousness were stabilized—in the domain of adaptive optimism—by a host of factors impinging on the brain-mind. These fac-tors range all the way from raw energy (in the forms of photons and heat) up to the most abstract internal constructs about our self-worth and our place in our social world. This makes all kinds of sense. But how does it work? What makes it fail? And if it does fail, how can we establish a new equilibrium?

The story of the discovery, development, and refinement of the anti-depressant drugs is one of the most exciting and informative chapters in the history of modern psychopharmacology. Because it is so directly connected to the model of sleep and dreaming, the biogenic amine theory of depression and the model of antidepressant action that supports it are also central to the development of the brain-mind paradigm's effort to account for clinically significant and desirable alterations in conscious state. To make a long story short, the same brain-mind energy control systems that regulate sleep and dreams appear to simultaneously regulate mood. But they do so on quite different time scales, a puzzling fact that needs our attention.

Activation and Modulation

So far we have treated activation and modulation as separate processes. We will want to preserve that distinction even now as we explore their close interaction. In mania, whether it be driven by stimulants or by high levels of endogenous aminergic neuromodulator, the activation level is raised and the tendency to sleep is lowered. In depression, whether it comes in response to amine depletion by drugs like reserpine or to low levels of endogenous neuromodulators, the activation level is always low and the tendency to sleep may be high. There are notable exceptions to these rules, especially in depression, which is sometimes associated with extreme motor agitation and severe insomnia.

In the discussion that follows we will focus mainly on norepine-phrine, serotonin, and acetylcholine, the three neuromodulators most carefully studied by depression and sleep scientists. The dissociations that may occur among those three systems and other important neuro-modulators like dopamine limit the value of the generalizations we can make today, but they nonetheless provide a solid grounding for the future work that will help us understand exceptions to the rules we can now lay down.

The Biogenic Amine Theory of Depression

The positive effects of the monoamine oxidase inhibitor isoniazid and the amine reuptake blocker imipramine were both discovered by accident. Isoniazid was being used as an antitubercular drug when patients' reports of elation led Nathan Kline to test and to demonstrate its antidepressant power. Ronald Kuhn had synthesized imipramine, a tricyclic molecule, as a possible me-too analog of chlorpromazine. When Kuhn found that it had little or no antipsychotic potential, he tried it out on depressives, and voilà! They got better. After a while, that is. As with isoniazid, imip-ramine's antidepressant action was evident only after one to four weeks of administration.

Both of these wonder drugs boost the synaptic efficacy of norepineph-rine and serotonin, but they do so in quite different ways. Isoniazid blocks the action of the amine degrading enzyme monoamine oxidase, allowing the released amines to stay longer in the synaptic cleft (because they are less readily broken down). Imipramine yields the same final result but achieves it by blocking the intracellular reuptake mechanism for the biogenic amines that were discovered by the Nobel laureate Julius Axelrod.

Serendipity—or chance discovery—is the scientist's best friend. The mentally prepared scientist, that is. As Louis Pasteur wisely stated, "In the field of observation, chance favors the prepared mind." Of course, entrepreneurial opportunism plays its part in this story, too, because the pharmaceutical companies that held the rights to these agents were able to mobilize both the clinical trials needed to demonstrate efficacy and the marketing machinery to make the drugs widely available.

The fact that all of these agents, acting in different ways, both improved depression and increased the efficacy of norepinephrine and serotonin made practically irresistible the idea the depression was mediated (if not caused) by a decrease in the efficacy of one or both of the biogenic amine modulators. This idea was already prepared in the minds of scientists who had observed that resperine, a drug that depleted the brain of its biogenic amines, often precipitated depression.

So in the hands of Joseph Schildkraut and Seymour Kety, the hypothesis became: decreased biogenic amine efficacy = depression. Its corollary was: increased biogenic amine efficacy = antidepression. So simple. So clear. So basically correct. But so incomplete. And so unsatisfying because (a) we don't really know how or why biogenic amine deficiencies develop in depression, and (b) we don't really know why the antidepressant effects take so long to kick in. The synaptic deficiencies, if any, must be corrected immediately, but the desired clinical consequences are not. What's going on?

Sleep, Depression, and the Biogenic Amine Hypothesis

We can predict whether or not a given patient is likely to respond well to an antidepressant like imipramine by how dramatically the alterations of sleep that are typical of depression are reversed. This fact has two important implications: first, it makes the delay more tolerable because a positive outcome is easier to anticipate than an uncertain one; and second, it means that there is more than a casual tie between the immediate sleep effects and the delayed antidepressant effect. Perhaps the link is even causal. How so?

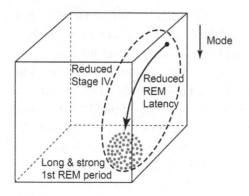

Figure 11.1
Depression. Depression results from decreased efficacy of aminergic neuro-modulation and reciprocal enhancement of the cholinergic system. Thus the set-point level of M declines. When subjects go to sleep they spend less time in stage IV and pass more rapidly to REM (seen as a decreased REM latency) and they spend a longer time in a more intense first REM period. When antidepressant medication raises M back up to normal levels, these sleep abnormalities disappear.

To answer this question we need to look more closely at the sleep side of depression. There are three parts to the main story. The first is that many depressives have a markedly reduced time to onset of the first REM period after falling asleep. This tendency to enter REM rapidly is measured as REM latency. The second part is that depressives may also have a marked reduction in time spent in stages III and IV, the deepest and most restful phase of NREM sleep. That could be one reason that their sleep is so unrefreshing. The third reason is that the first REM period is often longer—and stronger—than is seen in age and sex matched normal controls. These processes are represented in terms of the AIM state space model as figure 11.1.

What this all adds up to is that the forces that allow deep, energetically restorative sleep to occur and which normally hold REM in check are weakened. Thus REM occurs earlier, lasts longer, and is stronger than usual, all at the expense of deep non-REM sleep. That could be double trouble for depressives—they get too much of one good thing and too little of another!

We know the forces that hold REM in check—they are norepinephrine and serotonin, the same biogenic amines whose efficacy is compromised in depression. How satisfying! We now have one theory that explains three related processes: the daytime mood depression, the nighttime suppression of restorative sleep, and the nighttime REM enhancement. All three are the consequence of impaired aminergic neuromodulation. But there is more! From the other side of the reciprocal interaction model on which the brain-mind paradigm is built comes the recognition that aminergic weakness always denotes cholinergic strength. That's just what depressives don't need, because their increased REM propensity is driven by the same cholinergic supersensitivity that drives their depression.

So the worst kind of sleep for depressives is the kind they get a lot of: REM. That could be why REM deprivation temporarily lifts depression. And that could be why the antidepressants, especially the monoamine oxidase inhibitors (or MAOIs), work so well. They squash the overactive cholinergic system. REM deprivation does it for a day or two; MAOIs do it for as long as the drug is on board. Isn't that interesting! All of the reciprocities on the pathogenesis side of depression are mirrored on the therapeutic side. Let's fold the sleep and therapy facts into the integrated formula.

Aminergic weakness (and cholinergic strength) are associated with depression and its sleep abnormalities. Effective treatments for depression correct the sleep abnormalities by potentiating the aminergic system and by countering the cholinergic system. So far, so good. The problem is that these changes do not occur simultaneously. Instead, the sleep correction may lead the mood fix by days or weeks.

Long-Term Processes in Sleep and Depression

We are still embarrassed by our ignorance regarding the lag between treatment initiation and clinical benefit in depression. Can the fact that the sleep abnormalities are corrected first help us here? The fact they are corrected immediately—on the first day of treatment—could mean that the sleep architecture signs of depression are directly mediated by changes in synaptic efficacy. But this emphasizes the conclusion that the antidepressant effects cannot possibly be so mediated and demands that we consider downstream, intracellular processes almost certainly involving long-term shifts in cell metabolism. It is these energetic shifts that are definitive in the pathogenesis and the treatment of depression.

Recalling that the immediately visible correction of sleep architecture predicts the eventual reversal of depression, we can say that the synaptic level changes are necessary but not sufficient for antidepressant action. As soon as the efficacy of noradrenergic and/or serotonergic synapses is raised, larger amounts of the second messenger, cyclic adenine monophosphate (cAMP) are produced intracellularly. The second messenger eventually effects the transcription of genetic information which, in turn, instructs the genome to raise the production of gene products; the level of enzymes controlling cell metabolism is also raised. The converse is true of acetylcholine and its second messenger, cyclic guanine monophosphate (cGMP). That could mean that it is the proper mix and level of second messenger signals to the cells' own metabolic control system that characterizes drugs that are going to work.

What do we know about sleep and cell metabolism? Nowhere near enough. But there is some very clear handwriting on the wall that says good news may be on the way. First of all, we all know that in normal subjects sleep responds to fatigue and reverses it. Second, we know that sleep deprivation at first makes fatigue worse and then, later, much worse. Third, we now know that sleep deprivation is uniformly fatal if it is sustained for three to four weeks.

In other words, it takes about the same length of time to kill an animal with sleep deprivation as it does to cure a person with those drugs that restore sleep to normal for the duration of their administration. Some of those alterations are variations on the theme of sleep deprivation. The total suppression of REM by isoniazid and other MAOIs is a particularly striking example. Successful treatment of depression may thus depend upon pushing the two sides of the reciprocal interaction system to such extreme limits that REM sleep is impossible.

Are all of these parallelisms coincidences? To me it seems unlikely. I am impressed by the fact that the fatal effects of sleep deprivation all point to changes in cell metabolism that adversely affect energy flow and energy balance. Animals that die of sleep deprivation can't regulate dietary calories and so waste away, losing weight in the presence of limitless food that they devour in a vain effort to stay calorically even. En route to their demise they also become thermolabile; they are no longer able to defend their body temperature against heat loss in ambient temperatures that would not normally tax their regulatory capacity at all. Finally, they become so infection prone that they are overrun by bacteria from their own bowels, indicating a failure of immune system function. And again, all of these disastrous effects, which take weeks to develop, are immediately reversed by sleep!

The point of this argument-by-analogy is not to make a simplistic identity between the biogenic amine dynamics in depression/antidepression and REM sleep/REM sleep deprivation. To close that circle we would need to know the answers to such questions as these: Does sleep shift cell energy metabolism so that the costs of waking energy release are balanced? Does sleep deprivation make such restorative processes impossible? Does depression shift cell energy metabolism in the same direction as sleep deprivation? Over the long term, does antidepressant medication help restore the balance in the same way that normal sleep appears to? And, of course, what are the precise cell metabolic events that mediate the deleterious effects of depression and sleep deprivation? As sleep research crosses the threshold of molecular biology in the new millennium we can hope to learn more about the neural energetics of sleep and mood regulation.

Selective Serotonin Reuptake Blockade

Hoping to avoid such side effects as the sleep disruption and the occasional cardiac complications of the tricyclic antidepressants, and following the principle that clean drugs are theoretically preferable to dirty ones, the pharmaceutical industry has developed the selective serotonin reuptake blockers, a third generation of chemical agents to relieve depression.

In part due to successful marketing and in part due to remarkable public receptivity, these drugs have been widely prescribed not only for major depression, but also for obsessive compulsive disorder, anxiety, and just about anything a patient might report to a doctor, including wanting to feel more vital and enthusiastic about life. An only slightly exaggerated joke has it that New Yorkers today consider themselves to be at a competitive disadvantage if they are not taking Prozac! In other words, indiscriminate prescription has made these drugs so widely available as to beg comparison with recreational drug demographics. The distinction between the legal and the illegal is now so blurred as to make us realize that we are living in a drug culture on both sides of the law.

As the name implies, all of the SSRIs block the reuptake of serotonin, but not norepinephrine. Some, like fluoxetine (Prozac), are relatively free of anticholinergic properties, whereas others (e.g., paroxetine, known as Paxil) are as anticholinergic as some of the tricyclics. Unfortunately, all of these new drugs disrupt sleep at least as much as their predecessors and do so in a distinctive and problematic way that warrants our close scrutiny.

Here is the point: the SSRIs may well make us feel peppier in the daytime, but the cost is a blight on our sleep architecture that rivals the Russian bombardment of Grozny in Chechnya. True, the drugs don't kill innocent women and children, but they wreak such havoc with the eye movement control systems of the brain stem as to break down the walls between REM and NREM sleep. Like bombardment, the higher the dose fired on the brain, the greater the destruction of sleep architecture, until finally all of the walls come down!

Naturally, the propensity of SSRIs to strike at the heart of the REM sleep generator mechanism in the brain stem leads to all sorts of interesting and problematical effects on sleep and dreaming. But what is most alarming is the fact that some of the alterations in sleep architecture last for (now) up to a year after drug discontinuation! This cannot be a good sign, and it may well be a bad one, given our previous experience with antipsychotic medications like the chlorpromazine commonly known as Thorazine. As we have previously noted, those drugs caused Parkinson-like motor disturbances that could be partially reversed with anticholinergics, allowing patients to go on taking the drugs for years only to discover that other Parkinson-like motor symptoms—the dyskinesias mentioned earlier—emerged late in the game and persisted even after the drugs had been stopped. Apparently, the patients' motor systems are irreversibly altered. At what price altered states of consciousness?

Now I recognize that, even as I write, I will be called an alarmist and asked if I don't think the benefits outweigh the risks. So I'll answer that question right away. Yes, I do think the benefits are strong. But outweigh the risks? I can't yet say, nor can anyone else. But given the chlorpromazine experience, I think it is important to emphasize the risks early in the game so that they can be recognized by patients and their doctors, who can then decide together how to recognize and to minimize those risks.

Sleep and Dream Effects of the SSRIs

It is important to point out that basic sleep researchers make mistakes that are every bit as egregious and every bit as persistent as those of our clinical colleagues. From 1969 to 1975, it was widely held that serotonin promoted sleep. If that were true, then the SSRIs would be sedatives, not sleep saboteurs! In fact, there is paradoxical sedation in a very high percentage of users, but this effect is not easily attributable to the enhancement of serotonergic efficacy. So strong was the serotonin hypothesis that it worked its way into textbooks, where it lived for fifteen years after it had been clearly shown that serotonin was actually a sleep inhibitor and, reciprocally, a wake-state enhancer.

In the brain-mind, as in the marketplace, you never get something for nothing. The SSRIs exact the price of lightening sleep in exchange for enlivening waking. SSRI takers may have difficulty falling asleep and staying asleep, and they often say that they are dreaming all night long. Perhaps this is because of the increase in time they spend awake, but other explanations suggest themselves. One is an increase in stage I, the phase of sleep in which sleep onset and later night dreaming is so common, at the expense of stage II, which, especially early in the night, is devoid of reported conscious experience. Later in the night, stage II, which is normally associated with dreaming, may become even more oneirogenic because of the admixture of eye movements with it. Stages III and IV, already curtailed in depression, may be suppressed to even lower levels when the SSRIs are called to the rescue.

In terms of the brain-mind paradigm and its 3-D map, the AIM model, SSRIs produce the equivalent of a stimulant effect as well as paradoxical sedation. The upward shift of the M dimension, caused by the elevation in aminergic drive, makes descent into deep sleep impossible, just as amphetamines make falling asleep at all more difficult. Because subjects spend much more time in light sleep at or near waking levels, they naturally experience more dreaming *and* they are more aware of it because they awaken more often.

But that's not all. There's the REM enhancement effect, too. Serotonin plays an active role in the regulation of the brain stem saccade generator. This is the automatic brain stem system by which we make the continuous involuntary eye movements necessary to waking vision. This saccade system never shuts down completely and, in fact, there are always some eye movements in so-called NREM sleep. But with increasing dose levels of the SSRIs, the saccade generator is less and less likely to go into abeyance because serotonin inhibits the omnipause neurons that inhibit it. The result is that NREM sleep becomes more and more REM-like and sleep consciousness is more and more dreamlike! It's as simple as that.

Or is it?

SSRIs and the REM Sleep Behavior Disorder

"Did you ever see a dream walking?" asks the popular 1940s love song, "Well, I did." And so did Carlos Schenck and Mark Mahowald when they recorded patients with the REM sleep behavior disorder (RBD) in their sleep lab. In chapter 8, I described the dramatic emergence in the REM sleep of some middle-aged people of motor acts that bore a $1:1$ relationship to the subjective experience of dream movement.

Now Schenck, Mahowald, and others tell us that not only does SSRI treatment potentiate eye movements in NREM sleep, but that it may also potentiate dream enactment in REM sleep. In other words, SSRIs may induce the REM sleep behavior disorder! How does this work? In addition to releasing the saccade generator from inhibition, the drug appears to interfere with the spinal cord inhibitory mechanism that normally blocks the central motor commands that so convincingly animate our dreams but do not result in real behavior.

Although full-blown RBD is still rare, subclinical RBD is so common as to justify the supposition of a continuum of motor abnormalities, ranging from eye movement release phenomena (all subjects), through subclinical RBD (25 percent of subjects), to clinical RBD (2 percent of subjects) in the Schenck-Mahowald data. That may not sound like too high a price to pay for relief of depression or severe obsessive compulsive disorder, but remember, the signs and symptoms of RBD sometimes do not go away when the drugs are stopped. And remember, too, that spontaneous RBD is an early herald of Parkinson's disease. That doesn't mean that SSRIs will cause Parkinson's disease, but it does mean that we should be on the lookout. Forewarned is forearmed, and our warning comes from our experience with Thorazine, which also caused long-lasting motor effects.

In fact, the SSRI-RBD link sounds a lot like the Thorazine–tardive dyskinesia tie-in, doesn't it? What possibly common underlying mechanism
could unite these apparently disparate phenomena? One answer is dopamine, whose production by the substantia nigra is deficient in spontaneous Parkinsonism. Dopamine is blocked, hence rendered functionally
deficient, by the antipsychotics that produce both immediate and delayed
Parkinsonian side effects. Serotonin inhibits dopamine, which means that
potentiating serotonin with SSRIs could also render dopamine less functionally efficacious. Acetylcholine is in dynamic reciprocity with *both* serotonin and dopamine. Acetycholine causes an increase in dopamine's
efficacy in some circuits and a decrease in others.

The point here is the same one I have made over and over again in this
book. If you break into the Dream Drugstore, as you do when you take
either a street psychedelic or a medical psychotropic, you are likely to
experience impressive alterations in your consciousness and your behavior—some good, some not so good, some altogether bad, some immediate, some delayed, some very, very delayed, and some short term, some
long term, and some, who knows, irreversible. Be careful. Drugs are not
candy.

12

Psychosis and Antipsychosis: Opening and Shutting the Dream Drugstore

Psychosis is one of those frightening and unwelcome conditions that we hope only other people get. To be out of our minds is one of the worst things that can happen to us. And it can and does happen to many of us—or at least to someone in our family—all too frequently. Which of you readers has not had at least one family member suffer psychotic delirium due to Alzheimer's disease (there have been two in my family) or senile dementia (one more in my family), or psychotic delirium due to psychotic depression, mania, or schizophrenia (fortunately none yet in our case). Sooner or later all of us will want to know how to stop psychosis, or at least reduce it to levels compatible with social functioning.

By psychosis, I mean having hallucinations and/or delusions of sufficient strength and duration to interfere with normal wake state perception and cognition. And, of course, abnormally strong emotion is almost always associated with difficulty seeing and thinking clearly. So it follows that if I see or hear things that are not there and/or believe things that are not true, I am very likely to have unusually strong emotions. The one time that I myself had a sharply formed visual hallucination, I was terrified. And when I am very anxious—for whatever reason—I tend to misperceive and misinterpret other people's actions, even if I am not frankly delusional. The point here is that psychosis adversely affects our emotions and vice versa.

Those who can match or better my stories of psychosis know what I am talking about. Those who can't will readily realize that when they dream they too have psychotic experiences to help them appreciate just how unwelcome and disabling it would be to have them in the daytime. Dream psychosis is as florid as the most intense wake state psychosis by every standard: the hallucinations are totally domineering as they parasit-ize the visual, auditory, and sensorimotor perceptual domains; the delu-sion that we are awake and that our dream experience is real is seldom questioned; no matter how bizarre the dream events are, we accept them as real. One of the reasons for this impoverishment of insight is the verisi-militude of dream emotion; emotion is usually consonant with dream imagery and dream ideation even when dream images and dream ideation are not consonant with each other.

So you know what it is like to be psychotic, and you also know what a relief it is to stop dream psychosis if it's unpleasant, as dreams so often are! You are lucky. All you have to do is to wake up, which automatically shuts down the Dream Drugstore. By now you also know that waking up naturally reverses the neuromodulatory imbalance of the brain that is responsible for the psychosis of the dream, and so stops it.

The psychoses of major mental illness differ from each other and from dream psychosis in important ways that we should not ignore. The organic psychoses, so called because they are associated with chemical imbalances of the brain caused by drugs, alcohol, and nerve cell degenera-tion, are the ones that are most like dreaming. Hallucinations tend to be visual, and there are distinctive and severe changes in memory function that result in disorientation and amnesia. These changes do not occur in either affective (manic depressive) psychosis, or in schizophrenia. In terms of the Dream Drugstore concept, this means that there's something spe-cific going on in dreaming and in toxic delirium that the other psychoses don't have. My guess is that it is the extremely low levels of norepineph-rine and serotonin.

The psychosis of dreaming can nonetheless share delusional grandios-ity and emotional elation with the psychosis of mania. In mania, the hal-lucinations are more likely to be auditory than visual, as they are in dreaming. In mania, cognition is often tilted toward paranoia, but para-noia is surprisingly rare in dreaming. So too is the specific auditory hallu-cination of a voice speaking critically of us. Auditory hallucinations and persecutory delusions often go hand-in-hand in waking psychosis. Our immunity from them in dreaming should be instructive, but so far we don't seem to be able to learn a good lesson from it. Could it be due to the loss of self-reflective awareness? Or the relative weakness of auditory imagery? We don't know.

As for the psychosis of depression, with its ominous obsessions about death, disease, and stinking, rotting, or missing body parts, dreaming psychosis does, sometimes, come close. When we feel our teeth crumbling or imagine ourselves imperiled by dream damage and injury, we may be on the same psychopathological wave length as in depressive psychosis, but the volume is much lower. Why? One possible answer is that dream emotion, although often unpleasant, is rarely depressed. Anger and anxiety abound in dreams, but sadness, shame, and guilt are in relative abeyance. We don't even feel many of these emotions when the context suggests that we should!

The psychosis that least resembles dreaming is that of schizophrenia, because, like mania, it has the paranoia and accusatory auditory hallucinations (which dreaming lacks), and the emotional tone is often flat (about as far away from dream elation as we can get). Anxiety is about the only shared property, and that is not very specific. Perhaps it should come as no surprise that the typical schizophrenic psychosis is so different from that of dreaming. After all, it is the neuromodulator dopamine that has been most strongly implicated in the pathogenesis of schizophrenia, and that is the only neuromodulator that has not been implicated in dreaming. We will discuss this interesting difference in more detail when we consider how antipsychotic medication may work.

Dreaming and the Mechanisms of Antipsychotic Drug Action

When we awaken from REM sleep, we immediately terminate dream psychosis. The critical mediators of this antipsychotic effect appear to be the reactivation of the noradrenergic and serotonergic neuromodulatory system and the corresponding quenching of the cholinergic system. Why does this radical resetting of the modulatory systems change the state of the brain-mind from psychotic dreaming to sane waking? And can our answers to this question inform us about how exogenous drugs might work the same sort of magic?

The central idea here is that the neuromodulators set the mode of the brain-mind in two ways: one is by changing the pattern of regional activation, and the other is by changing the biochemical instructions to cells throughout the brain. I will review these two processes in terms of the psychosis-antipsychosis flip-flop.

In REM sleep dreaming, there is selective activation of the pontine brain stem, the limbic forebrain, and restricted parts of visual and multimodal association cortex. This activation pattern engenders psychosis by providing the brain-mind with the internally generated imagery and with the emotion that collaborate to constitute the psychotic dream plot. Two other processes also engineered by the state-shifted modulatory systems sustain dream psychosis: one is the active exclusion of sensory inputs that give the system external time-space-person data, and the other is the selective deactivation of the dorsolateral prefrontal cortex (which deprives the system of self-reflective awareness, insight, and executive guidance).

It is my hypothesis that this kind of phenomenological imbalance is characteristic of *all* psychosis. Put more succinctly: psychosis is promoted by the interaction of three factors: increased internal perception (1) and feeling (2), which work together against thought (3). A corollary of this theory is that a psychotic phenomenological imbalance is always the consequence of a changed brain activation pattern with facilitation of internally generated sensations and affects and a reciprocal disfacilitation of external inputs and executive cognition. Put another way, it is the collaborative interplay between external reality and internal reality evaluation that normally holds the perceptual-emotional generator system in check. When the balance between these systems changes, psychotic process becomes more or less likely.

REM sleep dreaming teaches us that one sure way to tip the balance in the direction of psychosis is to lower the efficacy of serotonergic and noradrenergic modulation. This allows the acetylcholine and dopamine systems to run unchecked, promoting internal perception and emotion modulation. Conversely, the switch to waking sanity restores noradrenergic and serotonergic control of the acetylcholine-dopamine axis; this chemical shift dampens internal perception and emotion generation in limbic and paralimbic structures while strengthening top-down control via the dorsolateral prefrontal cortex.

One general rule might thus be that good antipsychotic medications will be those that

1. increase serotonergic efficacy
2. increase noradrenergic efficacy
3. decrease dopaminergic efficacy and
4. decrease cholinergic efficacy.

Table 12.1
Interactions of Major Psychoactive Drug Classes with Neuromuscular Systems

	↑5HT	↑NE	↓DA	↓ACh
MAOIs	++	++		
Tricyclics	+	+		+
SSRIs	++			+
Neuroleptics			++	+

Table 12.1 is a scorecard indicating the neuromodulatory systems with which some of the major psychoactive drug classes interact. The table indicates that no one drug does it all, and that most are either 5HT-NE enhancers or DA-ACh blockers. Exceptions to the rule do not necessarily prove it. And in the case of the atypical antipsychotics, it is the antagonism to serotonin which may be critical to efficacy.

Neuroleptics, Dopamine, and Schizophrenia

The hypothetical link between dopamine and schizophrenia was forged by two reciprocally related findings. The first was that potent dopamine agonist stimulants like d-amphetamine and cocaine could cause a psychosis that was schizophrenia-like, in that it had auditory hallucinations and paranoia. The second was that the neuroleptic drugs that were effective in reversing both schizophrenia and stimulant-induced psychosis were dopamine blockers. Moreover, the antipsychotic potency of the neuroleptics was proportional to their binding affinity to the D2 receptor.

These foundational discoveries continue to underlie the succession of increasingly complex and sophisticated models of the pathogenesis and treatment of schizophrenic psychosis. Of the greatest interest to our effort to evolve a general theory of psychosis is the fact that dopamine-releasing axons project from neuronal sources in the midbrain to those forebrain regions that have repeatedly been implicated in dream psychogenesis. The mesocortical pathway connects the ventral tegmental area with the dorsolateral prefrontal cortex, an area known to be selectively deactivated in REM sleep dreaming. The mesolimbic pathway connects the ventral tegmental area to the nucleus accumbens of the limbic system, other parts of which are selectively activated in REM sleep dreaming. Significantly for our argument, it is the overactivity of the mesolimbic pathway that

mediates both amphetamine and schizophrenic psychoses. Also significant is the fact that experimental interventions that deactivate the prefrontal cortex lead to increased activity in the mesolimbic pathway.

We find that the models of stimulant-induced and schizophrenic
psychosis share three important elements: (1) facilitation of the limbic system, (2) reciprocal disfacilitation of the prefrontal cortex, and
(3) orchestration of these reciprocal changes by aminergic neuromodulatory systems. As it is item (3) that is causal in both models, we need to
examine similarities and differences in the neuromodulatory mechanisms
of the three classes of psychosis under scrutiny here.

Despite PET imaging evidence of activation of structures containing
them, there is no specific sign of increased mesolimbic dopaminergic drive
in REM sleep dreaming, but we do know that serotonin and norepinephrine modulate dopaminergic efficacy. This means that an indirect increase
in dopaminergic drive could be effected simply by shutting down the norepinephrine and serotonin modulation. The limbic system activation and
prefrontal cortex deactivation seen in REM sleep, stimulant use, and
schizophrenia might be a final common path to psychosis that can be
reached via different mechanisms, all of which result in a net enhancement of dopaminergic efficacy. The model would resolve the controversy
raised by Mark Solms's dopamine hypothesis of dreaming that we discussed in chapter 9.

Atypical and Typical Antipsychotics in the Light of the Brain-Mind State Concept

The nigrostriatal pathway connects the substantia nigra to the striatum,
an area important to movement. Substantia nigra damage leads to Parkinsonism, of which the REM sleep behavior disorder is a herald.

The first generation antipsychotics, now known as "typical" drugs,
were all D2 receptor blockers and, as such, very likely to produce Parkinsonian side effects. Because antipsychotic potency was associated with
D2 receptor affinity, it was assumed that dopamine overactivity was the
essential defect in schizophrenia and that a direct dopamine blockade was
the definitive route to treatment. But these drugs affected both the target
dopamine pathways of the mesolimbic projection and the uninvolved nigrostriatal projection. Unfortunately, that meant that movement disorders were the price that had to be paid for antipsychosis.

The effectiveness of the second generation antipsychotics (now called atypicals, because they have weak D2 blocking properties) show that this concept is not valid. Drugs like clozapine do not cause the Parkinsonian side effects even though they are very successful in terminating psychosis.

This surprising finding has forced the schizophrenia psychopharmacology field to recognize that psychosis is the outcome of interactions among several neuromodulatory systems, not a derangement of the dopamine system alone. That being the case, it is possible to act on dopamine indirectly with drugs that alter noradrenergic and serotonergic function in ways that simulate the dream antipsychosis effect of waking up!

To understand how this might work, it is important to recognize that serotonergic and noradrenergic neuromodulatory neurons tend to fire spontaneously unless they are inhibited. This is because they are pacemaker cells whose leaky membranes depolarize on their own. As a consequence, they are reliable suppliers of their modulatory molecules unless they are inhibited. But these cells also have another remarkable property: they self-regulate by means of direct feedback inhibition via recurrent collateral offshoots from their axons. These recurrent collaterals contact the cell bodies via autoreceptors that are often inhibitory.

Drugs like clozapine that block these autoreceptors can actually lead to an increased output of the modulators norepinephrine and serotonin because the pacemaker cells that produce them are disinhibited. In this way, they can exert a damping effect on dopamine and acetylcholine, as well as on each other. The point here is that a change from psychosis to sanity often involves putting the brakes on dopamine and/or acetylcholine. The best way to intervene chemically may thus be to simulate the natural system that converts dream psychosis to waking sanity. Puzzling exceptions to this rule still need to be explained. These include the deleterious effects of anticholinergic drugs (like atropine, which causes delirium) and the beneficial effects of antiserotonergic drugs which, by enhancing dopamine, reduce negative symptoms in schizophrenia.

The Developmental Model of Schizophrenia

Abundant evidence points to genetic risk for schizophrenia, but this propensity does not inevitably lead to the disease, and some people who are free of genetic risk may become schizophrenic. This means that the optimal conditions for becoming schizophrenic must be a byproduct of genetic risk plus environmental insult.

The best understood environmental insult is an early brain trauma that leads to impaired brain development. During the fetal and perinatal period, the brain is particularly vulnerable to restriction of its blood supply and its concomitant choking off of oxygen requirements. According to one hypothesis, as a consequence of early cortical development defects, subtle but handicapping cognitive defects become evident later, especially in puberty, when executive functions are instantiated in the dorsolateral prefrontal region. According to another hypothesis, the temporal lobe fails to develop normally, leading, again, to subtle but incapacitating problems with memory and emotional function.

The net effect is to push the brain in a very REM dream-like direction. PET studies of schizophrenic patients' brains show deficient frontal cortical activation *and* limbic overactivation. The working hypothesis of schizophrenia investigators is that psychosis results when the overactive mesolimbic pathway is released from deficient cortical control. This is formally identical to our hypothesis of dream psychosis: the dorsolateral prefrontal cortex is deactivated and the limbic system is hyperactivated.

To test this hypothesis, Daniel Weinberger made frontal cortical lesions in weanling rats and showed that the animals demonstrate anomalous behavior after they reach puberty. Antipsychotic drugs normalize by the anomalous behavior. Interestingly, the atypical antipsychotic drug clozapine is superior to the typical antipsychotic haloperidol in the animal model, just as it is in human schizophrenia. How interesting it would be to record the sleep of Weinberger's rats before and after the lesions were made and again before and after antipsychotics treatment. As far as I know, this experiment, which is difficult but feasible, has not been attempted. Even more interesting would be a study of the effect of Weinberger's interventions on the pattern of regional brain activation, but so far the use of imaging techniques to document experimental animals' brain activation patterns in sleep has been very limited.

Schizophrenia and the Cholinergic System

As part of the growing recognition that dopamine-only theories of schizophrenic pathogenesis are incomplete and in need of revision is a new look at the cholinergic system's possible contribution to the clinical picture. This revival of interest is spurred by recent findings that clozaril not only plays on the noradrenergic and serotonergic systems, but that it affects the cholinergic system as well. From the point of view of the dream psychosis analogy, the fact that clozaril's highest affinity is for the muscarinic receptor is of capital importance.

The reason for excitement about this finding is that it is specifically the muscarinic receptor whose experimental activation leads to massive increases in REM sleep when cholinergic agonist drugs are microinjected into the brain stem. No other class of agent is capable of such a spectacular enhancement of REM, and all of the evidence suggests that REM is, in fact, physiologically generated by the acetylcholine systems of the brain stem. That means that our own normal dream psychosis depends upon activation of the muscarinic acetylcholine receptor. As Edgar Garcia Rill has wondered, could the same process be involved in schizophrenia?

The ideas behind this question are not new and the answers are not yet clear, probably because of the complexity of drug effects and the intensely interactive nature of the intrinsic neuromodulatory systems. We should remember that from the earliest days of modern sleep research in the 1960s, studies showed that REM sleep parameters were normal in schizophrenia. This argued against the idea that increased REM pressure underlay schizophrenic psychosis and condemned the hypothesis to an early and perhaps premature oblivion.

On the psychopharmacology side, it was only a decade later, in the 1970s, that scientists considered an imbalance between dopamine and acetylcholine as a possible mediator of schizophrenic psychosis. The general idea was that the excessive dopaminergic drive rendered the cholinergic system less effective, so it needed bolstering by cholinergic drugs.

This notion resurfaced in the 1980s, when tests showed that anticholinergic drugs could both decrease the efficacy of neuroleptics in the treatment of the hallucinations and delusions and reduce the withdrawal, isolation, and lack of energy.

As in dream psychosis, the hallucinations and delusions of schizophrenic psychosis are referred to as "positive symptoms," implying an increase in excitability of the upper brain circuits mediating perception and its associated cognition. Anticholinergics can precipitate these symptoms in normal subjects who have overdosed on atropine, indicating that cortical acetylcholine levels must be high to support waking sanity, as well as dream psychosis.

In addition to the waking memory impairment as a direct dream psychosis equivalent of the so-called negative symptoms of schizophrenia and depression, there is an indirect link between them and depression via other characteristic symptoms: lack of energy, loss of motivation, social isolation, and withdrawal. Either allowing REM sleep or giving cholinergic agonists makes all of these worse. These "negative" symptoms of depression are the ones that take days to weeks to clear up after the correction of the sleep disorder. In this case, the indirect anticholinergic effect of the antidepressants works its wonders by first suppressing REM and later by restoring normal energy flow in the brain. Thus anticholinergic drugs have an energizing, stimulating, and socializing effect, indicating that they are in fact antidepressants.

The revival of interest in acetylcholine's role in schizophrenic pathogenesis is symmetrical to a new interest in dopamine's role in dream psychosis. Could it be that in both psychoses the coactivation of dopamine and acetylcholine systems is necessary but only sufficient if either the other aminergic systems are in abeyance (dream and depression psychosis) or the dopamine system overpowers the cholinergic system (manic and schizophrenic psychosis)?

This possibility could provide a strong foundation for a unified model that says that psychosis may result in waking if either acetylcholine is blocked (atropine delirium) or dopamine is enhanced (amphetamine, manic, and schizophrenic psychosis) and/or if both acetylcholine and dopamine are enhanced but noradrenergic and/or serotonergic drives are reduced (depression and dream psychoses).

Fixing psychosis via prescription from the Dream Drugstore depends upon restoring the appropriate balance among those four systems. Dream psychosis yields to waking sanity and depression yields to euphoria if both noradrenergic and serotonergic influences are increased and acetylcholine output is checked. Schizophrenia and manic psychoses yield to waking sanity if dopamine is blocked and acetylcholine, norepinephrine, and serotonin are enhanced so that they fall within normal limits. If serotonin is raised too high, so will be the mood, and mania may be precipitated. If dopamine levels are excessive, psychosis may be precipitated. All of this evidence shows that the chemical balancing act is as delicate and hazardous as high-wire acrobatics in the circus.

Glutamate and Schizophrenia

Glutamate, the primary excitatory neurotransmitter in the brain, depolarizes (excites) the postsynaptic membrane by its action at several different receptors. These are known as the NMDA, AMPA, and kainate receptors. Their names derive from the man-made molecules that mimic glutamate and so activate the glutamate-binding sites. The NMDA receptor hypofunction hypothesis of schizophrenia is the most prevalent cellular-level theory in the current literature regarding the etiology of this functional psychosis. This hypothesis is favored over earlier theories invoking dysfunction in only the aminergic transmitters (e.g., dopamine and serotonin) largely due to the comparison of effects among the different hallucinogenic drugs.

In normal subjects the hallucinogenic and anesthetic NMDA-receptor blocker phencyclidine (better known as PCP or "angel dust") and related compounds such as ketamine produce the negative symptoms (such as apathy) and cognitive deficits (such as memory impairment) of schizophrenia as well as the positive symptoms (e.g., hallucinations) that are also evoked by the aminergic hallucinogens (e.g., LSD, mescaline) and psychostimulants (e.g., methamphetamine) (figure 12.1). Moreover, glutamate dysfunction accounts for two other key features of schizophrenia, its onset in young adulthood at a time when glutamatergic inputs to the frontal cortex are maturing (by the process of myelination) and schizophrenia's deteriorating course, which is thought to be due to defects in the normal mechanism of neuron death (called apoptosis) which can be triggered by the overexcitation of neurons by glutamate at non-NMDA receptors. The brain contains its own endogenous substances such as *N*-acetylaspartyl glutamate which, under conditions of pathology or imbalance, can act on NMDA receptors in a manner analogous to PCP and ketamine.

The interaction of glutamate and its NMDA receptor with other brain neurotransmitters, including the aminergic dopamine and serotonin neuromodulators which are the main focus of this book, is very complex and only a few, simplified accounts of how NMDA receptor hypofunction

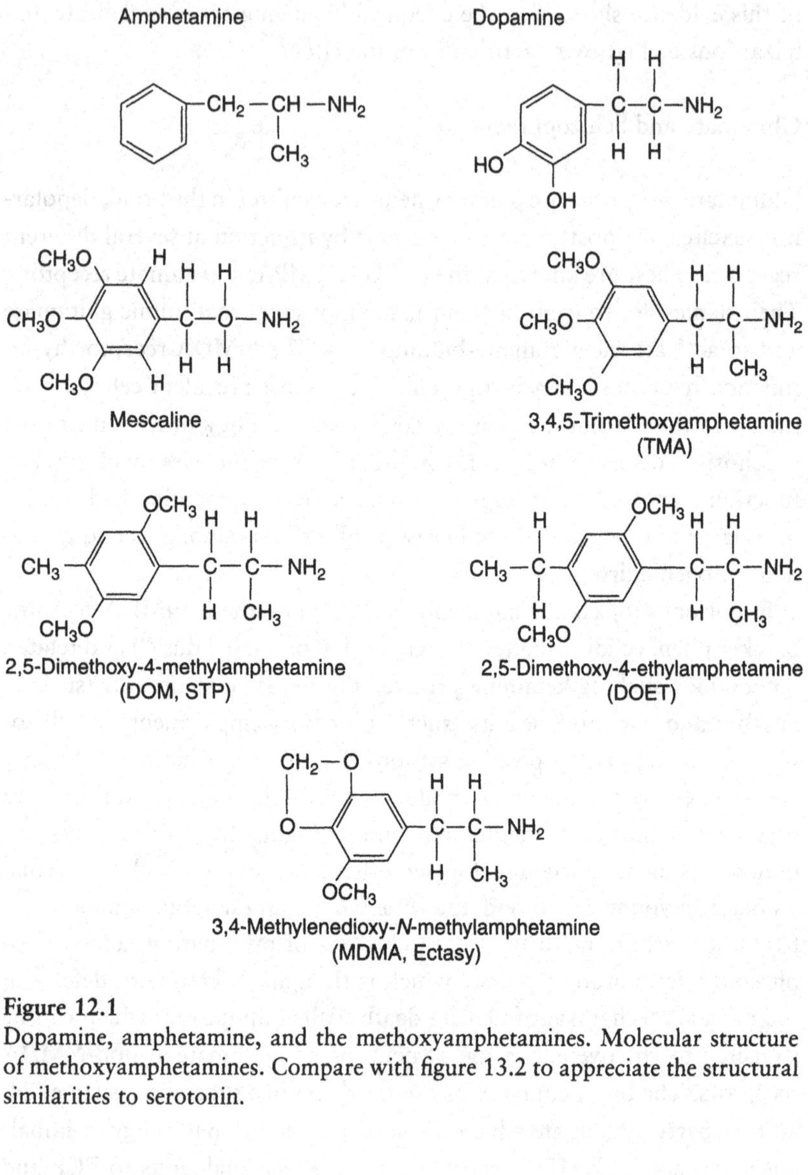

Amphetamine

Dopamine

Mescaline

3,4,5-Trimethoxyamphetamine
(TMA)

2,5-Dimethoxy-4-methylamphetamine
(DOM, STP)

2,5-Dimethoxy-4-ethylamphetamine
(DOET)

3,4-Methylenedioxy-*N*-methylamphetamine
(MDMA, Ecstasy)

Figure 12.1
Dopamine, amphetamine, and the methoxyamphetamines. Molecular structure
of methoxyamphetamines. Compare with figure 13.2 to appreciate the structural
similarities to serotonin.

might lead to the symptoms of schizophrenia will be described. In one model mechanism, NMDA receptors on neurons manufacturing the most ubiquitous inhibitory neurotransmitter GABA are defective, so that when they decrease firing, they release (or "disinhibit") other excitatory glutamate neurons from restraint and these, in turn, overexcite key portions of the cortex and limbic system (via non-NMDA glutamate receptors). This causes psychotic symptoms over the short term in normal subjects and, over the long term in schizophrenics. By the same mechanism it also causes excitotoxic neuronal degeneration.

Many theories on the role of glutamate and its NMDA receptor in PCP-induced psychosis and schizophrenia invoke intermediary steps that involve the aminergic modulators dopamine and serotonin. Glutaminergic hallucinogens may exert their effect by a secondary activation of dopaminergic systems. For example, in a recent model based on animal experiments, Torngny Svensson suggests that PCP and schizophrenia alter the balance and timing of dopaminergic input to subcortical ("mesolimbic") circuits relative to its input to cortical prefrontal ("mesocortical") circuits. In this model, PCP disrupts the intermittent, information-bearing type of dopaminergic input to the prefrontal cortex (which controls "higher" mental function) while it increases the mesolimbically projecting dopamine neurons' constant "noisy" firing pattern.

The link with serotonin includes recent studies showing that both the novel antipsychotics (e.g., clozapine and risperidone) and the indolamine (serotonergic) hallucinogens both affect cortical postsynaptic 5HT$_2$ receptors. A prominent researcher in this area, Franz Vollenweider suggests that "a dysbalance between serotonin, glutamate and dopamine in the limbic cortico-striato-thalamic circuitry may be critical to psychotic symptom formation . . . the neuronal substrate of normal and abnormal thought . . . is associated with a distributed neuronal network and with multiple interactive neurotransmitter systems." In support of this idea, Svensson has shown that the ability of the novel antipsychotics to correct the PCP-induced mesolimbic/mesocortical dopaminergic firing imbalance in animals may operate via both serotonergic and noradrenergic mechanisms. Another prominent serotonin researcher, George K. Aghajanian, suggests that the hallucinogens affecting the 5HT$_2$ receptors also have glutamatergic effects in the cortex, while the NMDA antagonists can also affect $5HT_2$ receptors indicating shared mechanisms between the NMDA and $5HT_2$ receptor hallucinogens.

Antiepileptics, Membrane Stabilization, and Mania

In discussing schizophrenia, we have restricted our attention to the rule of neuromodulation. A second general rule concerns the excitability of the brain with special reference to phasic activity of the sort that drives the REM sleep process (on the one hand), and clinical seizures (on the other). In chapter 9, I pointed out some of the phenomenological and physiological processes that REM sleep and epilepsy share, and emphasized the importance to both of temporal lobe activation.

Now we turn our attention to the antipsychotic potential of drugs that are also useful in treating epilepsy and speculate about the reason for their efficacy in controlling the affective psychoses, especially mania. Manic psychosis is formally like dream psychosis in its delirious aspect: we see the ecstatic elation, the grandiose delusions, and the poor judgment leading to social indiscretion in both states. Only organic delirium itself more closely resembles dream psychosis. What could account for these similarities?

The most obvious hypothesis is that in mania, as in dream psychosis with elation and grandiosity, it is possible to raise to very high levels the general activation of the brain and the specific activation of the positive emotion generator in the medial septum and other limbic regions. Because this effect can be artificially accomplished by taking amphetamines, it is reasonable to propose that excessive endogenous dopamine release (or increased receptor sensitivity) may be involved.

But whatever the neuromodulatory status of mania, it makes sense to reason that the exuberant positive emotion, emanating from a hyperactive limbic system, is unchecked by a relatively impoverished dorsolateral prefrontal cortex. Hence, the poor judgment and the disastrous social indiscretions are the result of takeover of the brain by parasitic internal stimuli just as occurs in epilepsy and in dream psychosis!

A clinical point of great relevance to our thesis is that mania is invariably associated with insomnia, meaning that one has lost the normal ability to shut down the noradrenergic and serotonergic systems and to run the cholinergic system unopposed. Thus mania is a kind of spontaneous sleep deprivation.

Now sleep deprivation also happens to be one of the most potent ways of promoting seizures. This is probably because the neuronal activity synchronization that is part and parcel of sleep is also part and parcel of generalized seizures. In other words, if one is well rested, one can hold in check an epileptic focus—like the spindle and slow wave generators of NREM and the PGO generator of REM sleep. This is undoubtedly the collaborative work of GABA and the aminergic modulators, especially serotonin. But increase the desire to sleep—by preventing it—and just as you increase the desire to generate spindles, slow waves, and PGO waves, you increase the ability of an epileptic focus to escape local control and take over the brain. In this sense, going to sleep is a bit like having a seizure, and staying awake is a little bit like having a manic episode!

Think about it. When you are "high" on booze, on drugs, or on sex, do you want to sleep? No. Do you feel elated, even somewhat giddy? Yes. Most of the neurons that exert local control throughout the brain do so by liberating the inhibitory neurotransmitter GABA; drugs that interfere with GABAergic inhibition, like penicillin, pentylene tetrazol, and strychnine, promote seizures. Drugs that increase GABAergic inhibition and/or otherwise diminish the excitability of local neurons are antiepileptic and their firing is moderated as much as it is modulated. A neuron can still fire appropriately (because the firing level is not depressed), but it can also stop firing rapidly (because feedback inhibition and/or intrinsic repolarization is prompt and effective).

In any case, it is easy to understand how something like "membrane stabilization" could help neurons be more temperate, and how a more temperate brain could more easily resist its own tendency to go wild. In clinical terms this means that such indulgences as flights of ideas, pressured speech, buying sprees, sexual promiscuity, drug taking, and manic psychosis will be less likely.

With these drugs the brain is not depressed as it was with the old fashioned sedatives like the barbiturates, and it is not sedated as it is with the benzodiazepines. The drugs simply keep it from getting too high and going out of control. By reducing the tendency for any local circuit to become anarchic, antiepileptic drugs act like neuronal policemen: no speeding, please.

How does it work? As with so many useful drugs, we really don't know. But the term "membrane stabilization" has a nice ring to it and brings the antiepilepsy and antimania forces into an understandable conjunction. It now appears that all anticonvulsant and antimanic drugs may have as their common mechanisms of action the damping of second messengers like cyclic AMP, which regulates energy dynamics inside brain cells. Every neuron in the brain has its firing propensity set by multiple mechanisms that converge on the cell membrane. The presence of drugs that either potentiate GABAergic inhibition or alter ion channel permeability raise the firing threshold of brain cells. They are thus less likely to go off half-cocked. Because hyperexcitability is like a wild fire that feeds on itself, fire in the brain is a very good metaphor for epilepsy and for mania. No wonder the membrane stabilizing drugs help control mania.

Here we are back again to the recognition that the brain has a great tendency to be plastic—to be permanently altered for good or for bad—based on its past experience. Whether that past experience be trauma (encoded as potentially conscious memory) or simple conditioning (recognizable as automaticity of distinctive behaviors), the brain keeps score, on time scales that range from milliseconds to whole lifetimes. Keeping score may involve adding up a propensity to mania via a fire-like process called kindling; or it may involve subtracting brain capacity, as in the hippocampal damage model of PTSD.

Have one seizure and you are more likely to have a second. Have one manic episode and you are more likely to have another. Thus the brain's ability to resist the excesses of epilepsy and manic psychosis are broken down by repeated attacks until one reaches a peaceful but not very pleasant endstage called, appropriately enough, "burn out."

Advocates of preventive treatment rightly argue that brain fires of epilepsy and mania must not only be rapidly extinguished once they begin, but even that people at risk should be treated with drugs to obviate the first attack altogether. There are two obvious problems here. One is knowing who is at risk; the other is the high cost of long-term treatment.

Who is at risk? For epilepsy, anyone who has had a concussion? For mania, anyone with a family history of mood disorder? If the answer is yes to either of these questions, we are talking very large numbers—maybe a third of the population?

How high is the cost? In financial terms, it depends on the ambitions of the drug companies and the stinginess of the insurers, both of which seem to increase exponentially. They could be changed, but it would take a social revolution not yet visible on our horizon. In personal terms, it's incalculable, because we don't yet know what will happen if we use any drug for 10, 20, or 50 years. I love the idea of prevention, but I am not excited about its immediate prospects!

Part V
The Recreational Drugstore

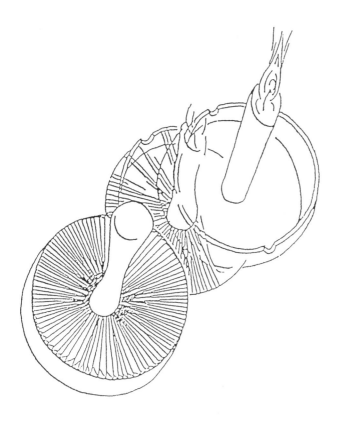

13

Good Trips and Bad: The Psychedelics

Psychotomimetics

All of the major psychedelic drugs have a close chemical resemblance to the neurotransmitters norepinephrine, serotonin, and dopamine.

—Solomon Snyder

Because the brain's state is controlled by neurons that exert their modulatory effects via chemical substances, it should come as no surprise to find that many drugs that alter consciousness without obliterating it exert their influence via interaction with the brain's own chemical control systems. Examples in this chapter include drugs that are not psychedelics per se such as the popular stimulants amphetamine and cocaine, which induce euphoria by their capacity to mimic the action of dopamine. Even narcotics, like opium and heroin, have stimulant effects that induce euphoria in parallel with their analgesic effects. In excess and/or after prolonged use, these initially euphorogenic agents can so unbalance the brain's state control chemistry as to result in delirium, the kind of psychosis that is quite reasonably thought of as a waking dream.

Interference with the serotonin system by big league psychotogens like mescaline and LSD can cause psychosis more promptly, and it is this capacity that made hallucinogenic drugs so popular in the 1960s. The psychosis produced by LSD is not, properly speaking, a delirium, but the fact that the drug acts via one of the major brain chemical systems involved in suppressing waking dreaming supports the general thesis of this chapter, which is that dreaming, delirium, and psychedelic states all share a common generic mechanism: a shift in the neuromodulatory balance of the brain from aminergic to cholinergic dominance.

Drugs that induce hallucinations and delusions are, by definition, psy-chotogenic. So is REM sleep. Following Snyder, the obvious hypothesis is that the drugs that are psychotogenic interact with the chemical neuro-transmitters that regulate the shift from waking to REM sleep. In this and subsequent segments of this chapter, we will examine the evidence for and against this hypothesis at the level of phenomenology, peripheral and central physiology, and structural biochemistry. I will then make an attempt to integrate the observations and evaluate the hypothesis. Al-though PCP is the common model psychotogen I have chosen to focus this section on LSD because it is possibly the best known, most commonly used psychotomimetic. It is also the most striking exemplar of the princi-ples of this book.

Albert Hofmann's LSD Trip

Q. When is a scientist not a scientist?
A. On Sunday!

This epigram summarizes the conclusions of my colleague, Jeffrey Saver, who spent the year between leaving Harvard College and entering medical school interviewing about forty of the world's leading scientists regarding the compatibility of their religious beliefs (their cosmic views on Sunday) and their scientific principles (their cosmic views on Monday through Saturday). When we alter our state of consciousness in the inter-est of spirituality, it is virtually impossible to retain the critical thinking and skepticism necessary to science.

Like so many of the scientists Saver interviewed, the Swiss biochemist Albert Hofmann (figure 13.1) was a believer in God. But in his case, we could alter the epigram as follows:

Q. When was Albert Hofmann not a scientist?
A. Never!

Even when he was out of his mind, Hofmann was capable of accurate self-observation. Hofmann is thus twice a hero. He resisted the impulse to interpret the visions that developed when he was synthesizing LSD-25 as either a visitation from the spirit world or as a spontaneous mental illness. Instead, he wanted to describe and investigate his inadvertent dis-covery with objective dispassion and analytic curiosity.

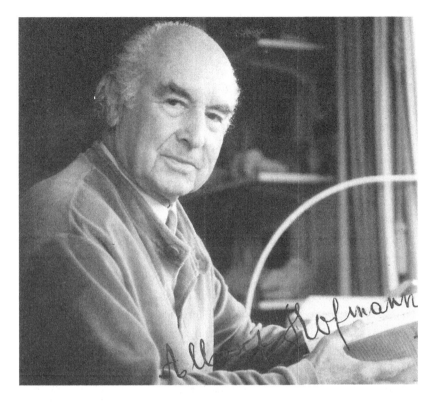

Figure 13.1
The Swiss biochemist Albert Hofmann discovered the hallucinogenic effects of LSD-25 by accident when he was working to synthesize molecules akin to ergotamine for the treatment of peripheral autonomic dysfunction. In a rush of what scientists call serendipity (or chance discovery) Hofmann realized that he had stumbled upon a far more important effect: LSD acted in the brain itself, altering its chemistry in the direction of psychosis and of dreaming. Descriptions of these effects upon his mind are given in the text. (Courtesy of the Albert Hofmann Foundation)

Here is the description of his subjective experience that he submitted to his chief, Arthur Stoll, following his first, entirely accidental ingestion of the drug:

Last Friday, April 16, 1943, I was forced to interrupt my work in the laboratory in the middle of the afternoon and proceed home, being affected by a remarkable restlessness, combined with a slight dizziness. At home I lay down and sank into a not unpleasant intoxicated like condition, characterized by an extremely stimulated imagination. In a dreamlike state, with eyes closed (I found the daylight to be unpleasantly glaring), I perceived an uninterrupted stream of fantastic pictures, extraordinary shapes with intense, kaleidoscopic play of colors. After some two hours this condition faded away. (*LSD: My Problem Child,* 1980, p. 15)

Note the equation of "an extremely stimulated imagination" with "a dreamlike state." From the facts that he "found the daylight to be unpleasantly glaring" and the corresponding release of "an uninterrupted stream of fantastic pictures," we can safely conclude that Hofmann's LSD visions were produced by a dreamlike shift in the chemical balance of his visual brain. And, indeed, Hofmann himself offered the hypothesis that the stimulating effects on his visual brain were caused by LSD's interference with serotonin, the brain modulator that later physiological studies showed to be radically reduced in REM sleep.

In making these sound conclusions, Hofmann was helped by the "kaleidoscopic play of colors" that is more typical of exogenously altered visionary experience than of the natural conditions of dreaming or psychosis. The dizziness suggested involvement of his brain stem vestibular balance system, as is common in intoxicated conditions. The brief duration of Hofmann's first psychedelic experience was another clue. In retrospect, this brevity was a function of the very minuscule amounts of drug that could have entered his body via his contaminated finger tips, either directly across his skin or through his mouth, which he may have inadvertently touched. Thus Hofmann immediately appreciated the extreme potency of LSD, a feature explainable only in terms of a highly specific interaction with critical control systems in the brain.

The more prolonged, severe, and distinctly psychotic experience that ensued when he voluntarily ingested 25 micrograms of LSD only three days later bore out Hofmann's hypothesis. As before, the drug initially caused anxiety, dizziness, and visual distortions, but now "symptoms of paralysis" and a "desire to laugh" were added to the mix, indicating effects on the postural and emotional control systems of the brain stem and limbic systems, respectively.

Alarmed by the severity of his symptoms, Hofmann asked his assistant to accompany him home, "by bicycle, no automobile being available because of wartime restrictions." Despite feeling that he could not move, he rode home rapidly without mishap. Then:

The dizziness and sensation of fainting became so strong at times that I could no longer hold myself erect, and had to lie down on a sofa. My surroundings had now transformed themselves in more terrifying ways. Everything in the room spun around, and the familiar objects and pieces of furniture assumed grotesque, threatening forms. They were in continuous motion, animated, as if driven by an inner restlessness. The lady next door, whom I scarcely recognized, brought me milk—in the course of the evening I drank more than two liters. She was no longer Mrs. R., but rather a malevolent, insidious witch with a colored mask. (*LSD: My Problem Child,* p. 17)

The visual delusions now share with natural dreams the sense of continuous motion that prompted us to characterize them as visuomotor rather than simply visual. This is an important point, because it supports the theory that both LSD and dream visions may have their origin on the motor side. This could be due to changes in the excitability and circuit dynamics of the oculomotor and vestibular control systems of the brain stem.

The negative emotions that became increasingly unbearable and made this LSD trip a bad one are also characteristic of dreaming; we can speculate that when serotonin modulation is impaired, either naturally (in dreams), pathologically (in depression), or artificially (in LSD states), the limbic lobe centers of dysphoric emotion are activated. And, as is true of dreaming, volition is impaired, the loss of voluntary control that Hofmann describes as follows:

Even worse than these demonic transformations of the outer world, were the alterations that I perceived in myself, in my inner being. Every exertion of my will, every attempt to put an end to the disintegration of the outer world and the dissolution of my ego, seemed to be wasted effort. A demon had invaded me, had taken possession of my body, mind, and soul. I jumped up and screamed, trying to free myself from him, but then sank down again and lay helpless on the sofa. The substance, with which I had wanted to experiment, had vanquished me. It was the demon that scornfully triumphed over my will. I was seized by the dreadful fear of going insane. (*LSD: My Problem Child,* p. 17)

Hofmann has now clearly moved into demonic possession country! With the dissolution of his will, his essential self has been split and a part of him replaced by an external agent, the demonic drug—shades of the devil that was thought to corrupt us by temptation; shades of the succubus that seduced men; shades of the incubus that seduced women in their sleep; and shades of the alien invaders that spirit some modern men and women away to other planets for bizarre rituals or unwelcome surgical interventions without their bed partners even noticing their absence. Indeed, Hofmann himself believed that he was outside his body as he reached the climax of his psychosis. This is dissociation with a vengeance!

Despite these derangements of perception and self-image, Hofmann had enough insight to call his doctor, but by the time the doctor arrived he could not utter a coherent statement, so his assistant had to give the history. As is so often the case in acute psychosis, there were no external physical signs except widely dilated pupils. Bed rest, but no medication, was prescribed, and on that regime the crisis passed. On the downslope, he could once again enjoy the psychedelic effects:

Now, little by little I could begin to enjoy the unprecedented colors and plays of shapes that persisted behind my closed eyes. Kaleidoscopic, fantastic images surged in on me, alternating, variegated, opening and then closing themselves in circles and spirals, exploding in colored fountains, rearranging and hybridizing themselves in constant flux. It was particularly remarkable how every acoustic perception, such as the sound of a door handle or a passing automobile, became transformed into optical perceptions. Every sound generated a vividly changing image, with its own consistent form and color. (*LSD: My Problem Child*, p. 19)

Note again that the visual imagery is geometric, not scenario-like as it is in dreaming. Although I have been able to induce kaleidoscopic imagery in my dreams by assiduous pre-sleep autosuggestion, they never arise spontaneously. This suggests that the visual autostimulation may be effective on a very early stage of processing, perhaps even the retina, as with the phosgenes the French self-experimenter Hervé de St. Denis and the American psychophysiologist George Ladd described. Contrastingly, recent imaging studies indicate that the brain activation of REM sleep is most pronounced in cortical associative areas, a much higher level of processing that is consonant with the scenario form of dream vision.

However, triggering visual imagery through auditory stimulation is clearly a central process reflecting a failure of sensory channel specificity called synesthesia. The most likely common cause of all these phenomena is impaired inhibition; a likely culprit is the interference with serotonin that results from LSD occupying its target receptor sites on brain neurons.

By late evening the LSD had left those brain receptor sites, and Hofmann was able to sleep. Sadly, Hofmann said nothing about his dreams, but did note that sleep completely cured his psychosis. When he awakened,

a sensation of well-being and renewed life flowed through me. Breakfast tasted delicious and gave me extraordinary pleasure. When I later walked out into the garden, in which the sun shone now after a spring rain, everything glistened and sparkled in a fresh light. The world was as if newly created. All my senses vibrated in a condition of highest sensitivity, which persisted for the entire day. (*LSD: My Problem Child*, p. 19)

We can't know if this post-sleep euphoria was a residual drug effect or simply relief at having recovered from the dreadful effects of his remarkable discovery. There must have been a rush of elation caused by the recognition that nature had just presented Hofmann with a gift as precious as Newton's apocryphal apple.

In Hofmann's case, it was a law of brain-mind gravity that was revealed by the blow to the head that LSD had delivered. If one alters the delicate neuromodulatory balance of the brain, the brain-mind can move out of its canonical trajectory through the state space and enter regions otherwise normally forbidden.

By 1980, the time that Hofmann wrote up his experiences, the role of the neuromodulators serotonin and dopamine in controlling conscious states was well established. Hofmann knew from the work of Gaddum and others that LSD blocked serotonin and enhanced dopamine transmission in the brains of animals, yet Hofmann stopped short of speculating about the possible brain mechanisms of his experience that he could have derived from that knowledge.

We can develop two very plausible and distinct hypotheses to integrate Hofmann's LSD story with sleep and dream research (on the one hand) and with schizophrenia research (on the other). Serotonin modulation provides the link to dreaming and dopamine modulation provides the link to schizophrenia.

Serotonin and Dreaming
Single cell recordings in the raphé nuclei of the brain stem show that the serotonin-containing cells are actively suppressed during REM, the stage of sleep most strongly correlated with dreaming. The serotonin system exerts a restraining effect on the acetylcholine neurons that actively and directly mediate the REM sleep events responsible for visual system activation and dream hallucinations. Thus when the serotonin system is suppressed, either naturally in REM or pharmacologically by LSD, the cholinergic system is released and visual hallucinations become more probable. The molecular structures of LSD and serotonin can be compared in figure 13.2.

Lysergic acid diethylamide (LSD)   Serotonin

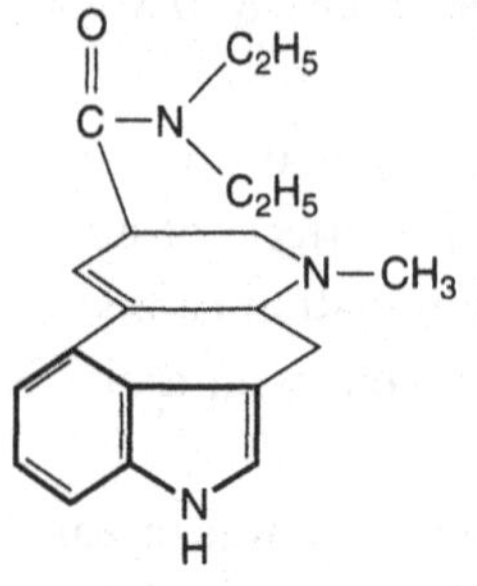

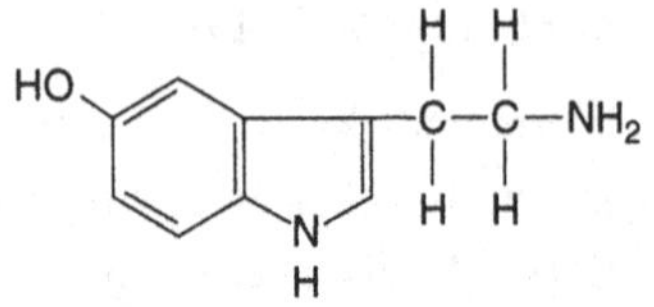

Figure 13.2
LSD and serotonin. LSD may exert its serotonin agonist and antagonist effects via the indoleamine molecular structure that both the synthetic and natural state altering chemicals possess.

Of course, there is an important difference between LSD and dream hallucinations: LSD images are often kaleidoscopic, whereas dream images are formed and scenario-like. And even though LSD causes an arrest of serotonin neuronal discharge, it does not enhance REM sleep. On the contrary, it promotes arousal both in humans and in animals, perhaps via the dopamine enhancement that links LSD to schizophrenia.

One result we could expect from these contrasting and partially antagonistic effects would be a dissociated conscious state with some aspects of dreaming (the visual phantasmagoria) occurring in hyperaroused waking.

Dopamine and Schizophrenia

The unpleasant aspects of LSD psychosis, and especially the sense of ego dissolution that Hofmann so vividly described, are reasonably ascribed to LSD-enhancement of the dopamine system. Based upon the strong correlation between the dopamine-blocking properties of drugs and their antipsychotic potency, scientists have long held that schizophrenia may be mediated by abnormal dopamine neurotransmission.

In Hofmann's account, other features of interest to the schizophrenia connection are the transmogrification of Mrs. R., the lady next door, who turned into a "malevolent insidious witch with a colored mask," and the grotesque threatening forms that familiar objects and furniture assumed. Such initial distortions, akin to the horrific images of Hieronymous

Bosch, are driven—as are bad dreams and schizophrenic hallucinations—by negative emotions, especially fear.

The shift in emotion from the not unpleasant sense of intoxication that accompanied the first, accidental ingestion, and the distinctly noxious, exclusively dysphoric feelings of the second, intentional one is, without doubt, a dose dependent effect. Subsequent psychiatric studies revealed that whereas euphoria was common in the 2–13 mg range, dysphoria regularly replaced it at doses above 25 mg.

Antidote and Recovery

The cure for dream psychosis is awakening. As soon as REM terminates, the serotonin system escapes from inhibition and modulates the visual system in favor of the undistorted processing of external data. As the LSD effects wore off, Hofmann slept deeply, thereby restoring the efficacy of his own serotonin neuromodulatory system. Too bad we couldn't have recorded that first recovery night to detect Hofmann's REM, measure it, decide if it was more or less intense, and even perform an awakening or two to sample his post-LSD dreams.

In 1943, the best antidote that Hofmann could come up with was milk, but milk is a no more effective antidote to LSD than it is against insomnia. By 1980, it was clear that chlorpromazine, the phenothiazine antipsychotic that began the psychopharmacologic revolution in psychiatry in 1955, could ameliorate LSD psychosis as well as schizophrenia. And this closes the dopamine circle. Because chlorpromazine blocks dopamine receptors, its therapeutic efficacy in LSD psychosis gives further credence to our hypothesis of its dopaminergic mediation.

Phenomenology

In general, the psychotogens cause a shift in the perceptual/conceptual balance of the brain mind. Perception heightens while conception weakens. This is exactly what happens in dreaming and in major psychiatric illness as well. Table 13.1 summarizes the phenomenology that we will examine and categorizes it as dreamlike or non-dreamlike. In the table and in the following text we use the same formal approach that has guided our work on the phenomenology of dreams. Of course, not all drug-induced psychoses are identical, and this approach ignores the vast

Table 13.1
Phenomenology of Drug-induced Psychosis and Dreaming

Phenomenon	Drug-induced Psychosis	Dreaming
Sensation		
Intensity	↑	↓
Synesthesia	↑	↑
Pain	↓	↓
Attention	↑↓	↑↓
Perception		
Eidetic Imagery	↑	↑
Body Image	↑	—
Emotion		
Anxiety	↑	↑
Elation	↑	↑
Aggression	↑	↑
Cognition		
Orientation	↓	↓
Short-term Memory	↓	↓
Intellect	↓	↓
Imagination	↑	↑

range of differences in content contained by the shared forms, but the striking homology between the natural (dream) and artificial (drug) states provides strong face validity to the comparison and this, in turn, validates the psychophysiological interpretations.

Sensation
Because external stimuli are actively inhibited in sleep, sensation is markedly reduced. That is why the increased intensity of visual stimuli and the altered form of visual perception that drugs like LSD induce cannot occur in the dreaming that is associated with deep NREM sleep. However, when dreaming occurs at sleep onset, such phenomena as synesthesia may become quite prominent because the sensory gates are still open. The visual imagery of dreaming may therefore acquire hallucinatory intensity and a bizarreness akin to the transmogrification of objects and people so common to drug-induced psychosis. A striking similarity between the two conditions is the relative anesthesia; this diminished pain sensibility is the more surprising given the prominence of the ominous,

threatening, and even mutilating scenarios of some dreams and some psychedelic fantasies.

Attention and Perception

Subjects report that while their attention is often seized—and hence sharply focused—by both drugs and dreams, they cannot easily shift their focus voluntarily. This shared alteration in consciousness is related to the marked shift in balance between the internal and external contributions to perception. Drugs change this balance appreciably and dreams change it markedly because external stimuli contribute so heavily to psychedelic perception and so weakly to dream perception.

That the excitability of the central visual system is enhanced in both states is suggested by reported increases in eidetic imagery—like the crystal clear bar of glycerin soap that I saw in my Roman bath dream last night. The failure of dreaming to alter body image and body feelings is another product of the denied access of veridical body signals to the brain in sleep. There is simply no body image to distort, and although most dreamers see the fictive dream world as first persons, they do not commonly comment on their own bodies. Even those dreamers who see themselves in the third person as actors in their own dreams fail to report somatic alterations. An important exception is the incorporation into dreams of bodily changes incurred by trauma or surgery.

Emotion

The three most common emotions described in dream reports, anxiety, elation, and aggression, are also commonly intensified by psychotomimetic drugs. The social conscience emotions like shame and guilt are underrepresented, as are the loss emotions like sadness, hopelessness, and helplessness. Bad drug trips are, like nightmares and bad dreams, characterized by unbearable intensifications of anxiety, fear, and aggressive feelings, by the absence of elation, and by the occasional intrusion of depressive affect with exaggerated shame and guilt.

Cognition

In the face of such strongly enhanced perceptions and emotions, it is little wonder that both drug-induced psychoses and dreams impair the ability to think, to reason, and to analyze logically. Orientation (the ability to accurately assess time, place, and person) is sabotaged by the expansion and compression of time, by distortions, transpositions, and misidentifications of objects, and by transmogrifications of personal attributes. Thus even close friends may change, switch, or borrow identities.

The main cognitive culprit (or victim) of this cerebral disaster is short-term (or working) memory, without the full benefit of which it is impossible to keep the mind on track. Despite the loudly trumpeted claims of revolutionary concept formation in dreams (e.g., Kekulé's vision of the benzene ring, Otto Loewi's acetylcholine experiment, and Swedenborg's vision of the Church of the New Jerusalem), most of the mental products are, at best, good fiction, and, at worst, gibberish. I hope I am not being either inaccurate or unfair when I opine that the nocturnal musings of one of my distinguished scientific colleagues fall into this category. Similarly, psychotogens promote other-worldly grandiosity, transcendence, and ah-ha insights that do not hold up to the light of day.

The reason for this illusory intellection is, of course, the enhancement of imaginativeness, of fantasy, and even of confabulatory power. Reality testing restraint is overwhelmed by the force of imagery and emotion that drugs and dreams unleash.

When we trip the good trip or dream the big dream, we are treated to the scenes of a "magic theater" and become witness to "transparent allegories." The more we notice this striking parallelism between drug- and dream-induced conscious states, the more we are tempted to compare the change in the collective consciousness of the 1960s to the change in individual consciousness that occurs every night in REM sleep. How far can we go with this analogy? Is it illusory? Or is it an identity? Did the Woodstock dream merchants inadvertently discover the key to the waking lock on dream consciousness? We need to turn to comparative physiology and to comparative biochemistry to answer these questions.

Comparative Physiology

A crucial consideration is that the most we could expect psychotomimetic drugs to do is to impose REM-like physiological conditions on waking, not convert waking to REM! This consideration has important implications for our conceptual approach to the comparisons and for the way we assess and interpret the similarities and differences that we see.

With respect to the conceptual approach, we are basically postulating that psychotogenic drugs drive the waking brain-mind in the direction of REM sleep dreaming, thus producing an "altered state" that is in fact a hybrid dissociation, having some features of waking (e.g., an upright posture, open eyes, open sensory and motor gates, high levels of activation) and some features of REM (e.g., diminished central aminergic efficacy, increased cholinergic efficacy, diminished frontal cortical power, increased amygdala and posterior cortical power, etc.).

With respect to the data and our interpretation of them, we cannot afford to identify and discuss only the findings that are congenial to the homology hypothesis, but we must also take especially seriously those that are not. This is not only the demand of equity and balance, but the demand of strategy as well. It is only the latter set of findings that offers us any hope of explaining the differences that make the two states non-identical.

In discussing the physiological similarities and differences, it is for two reasons convenient to separate the peripheral from the central neurophysiology. The first reason is that there are dissociations between them such that the periphery can be sympathetically activated while the center is either sympathetically or parasympathetically activated. The second reason is that the central changes are, in all likelihood, much more important to phenomenology because it is there that conscious awareness is elaborated and because the state of the periphery may have little (waking) or no (REM sleep) impact upon central state.

Peripheral Physiology

Psychotominetic drugs tend to enhance peripheral autonomic changes mediated by the sympathetic nervous system. As shown in table 13.2, many but by no means all of these changes are also seen in REM sleep.

The exactly opposite effects of drugs and dreams on pupillary aperture and reflex excitability are important examples of informative differences between the two states. REM sleep is off-line—that is, the brain is dissociated from inputs and outputs—precisely because access of afferent stimuli to the CNS is blocked (e.g., pupillary myosis), as is access of internally generated motor commands to the peripheral muscles (e.g., inhibited deep tendon reflexes). Were this not the case, REM sleep would be waking (or a hybrid state even more like drug psychosis). And if the converse were

Table 13.2
Sympathetic Nervous System Changes

	Psychotogens	REM Sleep
Phenomenon		
Pupil	Mydriasis	Myosis
Cardiovascular		
Heart rate	↑	↑
Blood pressure	↑	↑
Thermoregulatory capacity	?	↓
Body temperature	↑	—
Reflex excitability (DTRs)	↑	↓↓

not the case, drug psychosis would be even more like REM sleep dreaming than it already is!

The other changes suggest a similar shift toward sympathetic activation. In Aserinsky and Kleitman's first published description of REM sleep (*Science*, 1953), they reported that heart rate and respiratory rate both increased. Soon thereafter, Frederick Snyder showed that systolic blood pressure also increased, sometimes to alarming levels, in REM. Psychotogens raise heart rate and blood pressure, too.

An obvious question arises: do these peripheral sympathetic activations reflect direct effects of the drugs on the peripheral autonomic nervous system, or are they secondary to the central effects? Although we cannot rule out a contribution from the direct route, a central contribution seems very likely for the following reasons.

First, changes in body temperature must reflect a central process, because body temperature is regulated centrally. To produce hyperthermia, psychotogens must somehow enhance sympathetic drive and/or block cholinergic drive on the thermoregulatory centers of the hypothalamus.

Second, we can compare this hypothesis with the well-known fact that body temperature declines at sleep onset but then remains constant in REM despite a complete loss of central thermoregulatory reflex response in that state! Because aminergic demodulation characterizes REM, it precludes a rise in body temperature (unless ambient temperature were suddenly to rise). The strong central cholinergic activation of REM may contribute to the loss of thermoregulatory reflex responsiveness in that state.

Third, in REM sleep, at least, it is a well-established fact that the tonic increases in heart rate and blood pressure are associated with brain stem mediated activation and that the dramatic phasic blood pressure and heart rate increases are correlated with the clusters of eye movement that periodically punctuate each REM period, whereas heart rate pauses occur in the inter-REM intervals.

Now we confront a puzzling paradox—how can a central brain state characterized by cholinergic (parasympathetic) activation and aminergic (sympathetic) deactivation lead to sympathetic activation in the periphery? Resolving this paradox might help us understand a corollary question: how can psychotogenic drugs that block central aminergic processes lead to peripheral sympathetic activation? We will see that the answer to both paradoxes is the same: there is a dissociation in both REM and drug-induced psychoses between the normal wake state correspondence between the central and peripheral autonomic systems. Central aminergic demodulation mediates this dissociation in both states.

Central Aminergic Demodulation in REM Sleep and Psychotogenic Drug Induced States

LSD first became available for experimental use at about the same time that work on the mechanisms of REM sleep came under scientific scrutiny. Based upon casual reasoning, some predicted that because LSD produced psychotic states, the drug would increase REM sleep and dreaming. But just the opposite happened. Pre-sleep administration of LSD resulted in a dose dependent suppression of REM and a reciprocally marked increase in waking. This experimental insomnia matches the insomnia reported clinically.

What is going on here? Are the analogies that constitute the premise of the LSD-dream enhancement hypothesis wrong? Or is there some other explanation? The answer to the second question is yes, which may mean that the answer to the first question is no and that the central idea of this book is valid. Let's take a look at the evidence for a shared mechanism that will help us understand why LSD makes waking more dreamlike while it suppresses REM sleep and normal dreaming.

From the earliest investigation of its physiological actions upon the heart of the sea clam, *Venus Mercenaria,* LSD appeared to interact with the synaptic action of serotonin. More specifically, it occupied serotonin receptors, producing enhancement of serotonergic action at some and blockade at others. If serotonin was a sleep mediator, the receptor action of LSD might well lead to insomnia or hypersomnia, depending on the net balance of its effects on different receptors.

Further study of the role of serotonin in sleep mediation led to the discovery that its release in the brain was actually highest during waking and that sleep onset was consistently correlated with decreased release. In fact, the decrease in serotonin release was continuous and progressive throughout NREM sleep, reaching its lowest levels at REM sleep onset. Sometimes 5HT-containing cells stopped firing altogether in REM.

What this means is that serotonin acts to promote waking, in part by preventing the intrusion of REM physiology into that state! To the extent that LSD interfered with this inhibitory role, it might therefore enhance the occurrence of REM-like phenomena in waking. Hence the hallucinatory changes in visual perception might be due to an interference with serotonergic suppression of endogenously generated imagery, and the increased emotionality could likewise spring from release of limbic emotion generators normally quelled by serotonin. Because serotonin also modulates the frontal lobes, the magical thinking, poor judgment, and intellectual deficits might again flow from LSD's effects upon neuromodulation in that structure.

All of these hypotheses about LSD and serotonergic transmission involve the nerve endings in far-flung regions of the forebrain. What about the brain stem itself? At about the same time that the sleep-wake serotonin connection was being made, an epochal discovery described LSD's effects on the serotonergic neurons of the dorsal raphé nucleus of the anterior pons in rats. To make a long story short, the drug turned them off, just as if they were in REM sleep, but the test rats did not go to sleep. This raised the possibility that LSD caused a REM-like serotonin demodulation of the brain in a waking animal. Here we have an example of dissociation at the molecular level!

We scientists are never satisfied even by data that fit our hypotheses very well. Why, for example, are subjects on LSD hyperaroused? Wouldn't we expect them to be sleepy if they suddenly had their raphé nuclei shut down? The answer to that question depends upon whether 5HT actually promotes all aspects of waking or just some, like the balance of internally and externally engendered imagery, or emotionality, or cognitive rationality. If this were so, then we could have waking with some specific subqualities suppressed but with others enhanced (like vigilance, elation, and poetic transparency). That's exactly what happens when we take LSD, and that's precisely what some folks like about it!

From a theoretical point of view, the idea that interfering with serotonin neuromodulation affects just some conscious state functions and not others has several important implications. First and foremost, it nails down the somewhat vague and unsatisfying notion of altered states of consciousness by specifying what aspects of consciousness are altered and by pointing to a specific mechanism for those alterations.

Second, it underlines the importance of viewing consciousness as a highly plastic, multivariate, dynamic function with an almost infinite set of possible instantiations. Third, it vindicates the comparative approach by showing that features of one canonical state (e.g., dreaming) can appear in another canonical state (e.g., waking) simply by changing one aspect of the control systems of the brain that normally maintain the discreteness of those states.

From a more practical point of view, the specification of the psychology and physiology of conscious state alteration by psychedelic drugs fully justifies the paradigm of model psychosis. At the same time, it naturalizes the model psychosis concept by demonstrating its continuity with normal dreaming, the most ordinary, banal, and easily studied model psychosis of them all! Most significant of all is the set of specific guidelines provided to those who prefer to alter consciousness away from the psychotic/delirious dream domain of the brain-mind state space. That should be all of us, but it is especially those mentally ill people who now have little choice in the matter!

Comparative Biochemistry of Psychotogens and Neurophysiology of the Serotonin System

The serotonin system of the brain, like other neuromodulatory systems, has its cell bodies centrally localized, projects its widely ramifying axons throughout the brain, and interacts with its postsynaptic targets via a wide array of receptors. The serotonin neurons are localized in the raphé nuclei of the brain stem and have three physical features that contribute to their function as reliable mode setting elements for the waking brain. Feature one is their pacemaker property, determined by a constant membrane leakage that causes them to spontaneously depolarize and to discharge continuously and regularly unless they are inhibited. Feature two is autoinhibition, determined by their dense local synaptic contacts with each other within the confines of the raphé nuclei. Feature three is their small size, which confers low conduction velocity upon their axons. The net result of these three features is a strong tendency for the whole system to fire in concert at a low regular rate and hence to guarantee a vast postsynaptic domain of a steady supply of serotonin.

This highly desirable attribute confers a constancy of biochemical operating conditions to neurons throughout the brain. It is the very essence of neuromodulation. Impulse traffic can rise and fall in classical sensorimotor pathways without changing the uniform background conditions that give states such defining characteristics as activation level, information source control, and information processing mode. The reason that the LSD-like psychotomimetics are so effective may be related to the fact that they all share the indole ring structure of serotonin itself and can then substitute themselves for the natural neuromodulator in the serotonin receptor (see figure 13.2).

These physical features also contribute to the dramatic susceptibility of the system to functional disruption by drugs like LSD. For example, even minute amounts of drugs with a high affinity for the autoreceptors of the raphé neurons can shut the system down quickly and completely. This is because they mimic the autoinhibition coming from neighboring raphé neurons and because this drug induced autoinhibition is constant and long-lived, not intermittent and short-lived (as is the physiological firing related autoinhibition). Thus instead of being reliably available, serotonin suddenly becomes reliably unavailable.

If serotonin release were completely blocked by LSD's effects on raphé neuron autoreceptors in human subjects, it hardly matters that LSD also blocks the receptors of its non-5HT neuron receptors throughout the brain. But, in fact, we do not know if the psychotogenic doses used by humans are potent enough to completely shut down the raphé system (or even if the human raphé neurons are as significantly slowed by LSD). Therefore, it is important to recognize that automodulatory effects could also be achieved via synaptic blockade in target neurons of say, the limbic and visual systems, as well as by closing off the source of supply in the raphé. We would expect the two effects to be additive.

Serotonin's effects include classical neuronal inhibition, as well as modulation. The study of dreaming teaches us that disinhibition is likely the cause of positive signs of hallucination, emotional intensification, and confabulation, whereas demodulation more likely causes the negative signs such as memory loss, disorientation, and bizarreness. Serotonin blockade induced disinhibition is one of the mechanisms by which the very same set of aspects of model psychoses is generated: the visual distortion and hallucination could result from visual system disinhibition; the emotional intensification could result from limbic system disinhibition; and confabulation could result from associative cortex disinhibition.

14

Feeling No Pain: The Narcotics

Sleep is a natural anodyne. Our dreams are surprisingly devoid of pain unless we are having real pain that intrudes on them. This analgesic effect could be simply due to a nonspecific anesthesia consequent upon the general lowering of consciousness associated with sleep. But the narcotic effect clearly indicates that there must be more to it than that. Dream consciousness, although entirely fictive, is vivid and often filled with unpleasant emotions like anxiety, fear, and rage. In fact, dreams conjure up violent scenarios in which the dreamer is chased, caught, beaten, shot, and even knifed without feeling pain. To explain this dream-related anesthesia we need to evoke either a failure to simulate pain or its active suppression.

A Sneak Attack

Painless knifings may occur in waking as well as in sleep. My colleague, Ralph Lydic, was the "Bantam Doc" mentioned in a front page story that the *Boston Herald* ran about the three young marine recruit muggers that he successfully repulsed by carving them up with his Swiss Army knife! The marines, although seriously wounded, didn't feel a thing, probably because the excitement of their attack released endogenous opiates from their brains.

Although those butchered gyrenes may well have been partially anesthetized by the alcohol that contributed to their bad judgment in choosing Ralph as a victim, they were not asleep. And they certainly weren't sleepwalking when they stalked him on Brookline Avenue as he made his way home from the lab after one of his late-night experiments. For Ralph, the awareness that his three assailants-to-be were coming closer and closer to him—even as he quickened his own step to elude them—was a feeling previously known to him only via his run-for-your-life nightmares. In the classic chase dream, apprehension turns from anxiety to panic, and finally to pure terror as we realize that we can't move our legs quickly enough to carry us to safety. And then we are caught, just as Ralph was. Usually we wake up at that point, and the violent scenario ends. Ralph didn't have that luxury.

As the *Herald* article pointed out, the three marine recruits were local boys, home on leave from Camp Lejeune, where they were being trained for mortal combat encounters in some far-flung jungle. Now the softball field they dragged Ralph into to rough him up is no far-flung jungle, and although three against one might be fair in war (where all is fair!), it's not fair in peacetime! Had Ralph been a guerrilla espousing some more threatening cause than sleep neurobiology, the marine thugs might have expected him to be armed and dangerous. But they never guessed that their diminutive victim was carrying a well-honed jackknife blade in his pocket and was ready to use it.

In the ensuing melee, their initial success in subduing Ralph misled them even more. Although they quickly pinned and pummeled him, Ralph was able to get out his weapon, open it, and begin to slash and thrust it about with damaging effect. He heard one of them say, "He must be hurt, there's blood all over the place. We better get out of here." Then they fled.

When Ralph got back to a street light, he could see lots of blood, but was relieved to see that he himself was uninjured. He quickly called the police, told them about his adventure, and suggested that his assailants might be wounded. As indeed they were! When they were arrested by a security officer on the Boston subway, one had superficial lacerations, one a pneumothorax, and the third a severed biceps! The wounds were so extreme that their lawyer got them off the DA's indictment by agreeing to drop their own aggravated assault countercharges against my colleague! It's a bit like the Bernhard Goetz case in the New York subway. If, in defending yourself from gratuitous attack, you gravely wound your attacker, the scales of justice may rapidly swing away from you.

Endogenous Analgesia

Had they been wounded by a landmine blast in Southeast Asia instead of by a disadvantaged knifer on Lynch Field in Brookline, a medic would probably have given these three kids morphine for pain relief. The amount of morphine needed would have varied according to several factors, including their emotional state, the severity of their wounds, the meaning of their wounds, and their drug histories.

Endogenous Opiates

It is hard to believe that one could have a severed biceps muscle and not notice it, but when fighters are pumped up they can take inordinate punishment without pain. The arousal system that normally keeps us awake keeps us ultra-awake when we are after someone or when someone is after us. This hyperarousal can be associated with elation if we are the predator or with fear if we are the prey. In the heat of battle either of these emotions can be exchanged for the other, or mixed, or be accompanied by rage, depending on the strategy we adopt.

Ralph Lydic, in fear, chose flight. Trapped, he turned to fight. Because he was not just playing games, his fight was both motivated and directed. Kill or be killed. I know the feeling. When I myself was jumped by three junkies behind my apartment and was being stomped after having been flattened by a nose-crushing left hook, I remember thinking, "These guys would just as soon kill me." The very thought pumped my modest physique into full emergency force. As I struggled to my feet with two thugs on my back, I said to myself, "This can't be happening," meaning I never knew I had such strength. And I never realized that my nose was blasted to smithereens until I ran up the alley, with my attackers in full pursuit, and tried unsuccessfully to stop the passing cars for help and saw the drivers' horrified faces as they sped away from me. When I reached up to where my nose had been, I felt nothing but bloody mush! But still I felt no pain! The pain only came, and then in unprecedented intensity, when the surgeon tried to put my dislocated turbinate bones back into place at the base of my skull.

At moments of survival crisis, the brain is awash in emergency levels of wake state neuromodulators (like dopamine from the ventral tegmental area or norepinephrine from the locus coeruleus), emergency hormones (like corticotropic releasing factor from the infundibulum and ACTH from the pituitary gland), and short-acting pain killers (like the enkephalins and endorphins), all of which put action-in-the-service-of-survival above the protective deterrent of pain or fear of pain.

Although actual occurrences of interpersonal violence are the very essence of nightmares and of post-traumatic flashback dreams, we are as far from dreaming as we could be in three important senses: (1) we are not paralyzed (so we *can* really flee or fight effectively); (2) we are hyper-cognitive (so we can invent biological strategies on the fly or—on the ground, as in these two cases); and (3) we form richly detailed memories (so we will never forget the danger or the survival strategy). Even though I myself was not the victim, I can't go by the Lynch playground without remembering Ralph's heroic struggle, his vengeance, and his escape. And whenever I see a stranger approaching me in that area of town, I cross the street!

The pain killers that the brain emits in these crises are called enkephalins (because they are in the head) or endorphins (because they are endogenous morphine-like chemicals). They occupy the same receptors as morphine and they trigger the same energizing second messenger (cyclic AMP), but because they break down more rapidly, their effects are more short-lived than exogenous morphine-like agents (such as heroin and morphine itself). Might they be released by the brain in the fictive emergencies of REM sleep? We don't know, but as other major hormones are released in sleep, it is not impossible.

A Rush of Elation

When a marine in Vietnam takes heroin on the streets of Saigon or is given morphine by a medic in the jungle, he gets more than momentary analgesia. Especially in the case of heroin, he may get a rush of elation, a feeling of well-being, and even of invincibility that is the perfect antidote to his chronic depression (because he is separated from his loved ones), his moral malaise (because he is fighting a losing war that many consider pointless), and his fear (because he could be wounded or killed on his next round of field duty). The stimulant-like euphoric effects of the narcotics are thought to be mediated by the norepinephrine that the locus coeruleus liberates, but it is obvious from the fact of dream elation that we can have euphoria even when the locus coeruleus is shut down! An alternative mechanism for euphoria is an increase in dopamine release in the nucleus accumbens (mediated by opiate receptors on the GABAergic controllers of dopaminergic neurons in the ventral tegmental area).

The legal and medical sequelae of Ralph Lydic's encounter with the marine recruits kept all four of them awake all through that fateful encounter night. But even these environmental effects acted through the brain's waking mechanisms, including the locus coeruleus and the hypothalamus, so they didn't dream *that* night. Only when they were safe enough—and unstimulated enough—were the brain healing and long-term memory enhancing processes mediated by acetylcholine unleashed.

Then and only then could the protagonists integrate real life events into their permanent cognitive and behavioral repertoires. In order for that to happen, the brains had to get over having been put on emergency hyperalert so that they could enter their maintenance mode—which is also pain free, hyperemotional, and wildly motoric. So phenomenologically similar are the on-line waking survival and off-line dream rehearsal states as to demand functional reconciliation. My intuitive hypothesis is that we are so well prepared by our dreams for fight and flight that when real life situations demand such action we can deliver it. Moreover, when real life demands and gets such responses, our dreams integrate the salient experience data into their protective matrix so that the next response will be even more effective.

The Battlefield of Everyday Life

Many urban landscapes are reasonably compared to war zones. When the threat of life-taking violence is omnipresent, even the innocent citizen is imperiled. Consider the Diallo case: the police gunned down an Ethiopian immigrant who moved his hand when told to "freeze." Drive-by shootings, stakeouts, and Mafia-style executions are now so commonplace in many inner city neighborhoods that mistakes are frequent.

One response to living in constant fear is taking drugs. Fanning the flames of fear to inferno heat is drug traffic. The current street drugs of choice are stimulants like cocaine, and the narcotics like heroin, whose sleep and dream link to the psychedelics we now explore. This link long antedates the postindustrial urban slum and the sleep neuroscience revolution. Like its modern psychedelic cousins, the molecules that can now be so easily cooked up in amateur chemistry labs and sold on the streets in plastic envelopes were derived from plants used in ritual practices.

The discovery that poppy extracts could induce euphoria, lethargy, somnolence, and dreamy stupor was made at least four thousand years ago. In Greek mythology, Nyx, the goddess of night, was a dispenser of opium poppies. One of Nyx's sons was Hypnos, the Greek god of sleep, and another was Thanatos, the god of death. Night, sleep, and death are thus all first degree relatives in the Greek imaginative mind.

All three conditions—darkness, mental obliteration, and somatic annihilation—are associated with the states induced by poppy extract, as well as those associated with natural sleep. So, too, are inspired transports of dreams. Coleridge and many of his romanticist brethren used opium to enhance the hyperassociative visionary processes that fed their poetry. Just as Nyx (the nocturnal poppy dispenser) begat Hypnos (sleep), Hypnos begat Morpheus (human dreams), Icelus (animal dreams), and Phantaseus (inanimate dreams, whatever they might be!).

It was Morpheus, the god of human dreaming, that gave his name to the chemical substance morphine, which was first purified from opium by the German chemist Friedrich Sarturier in 1805, precisely the time that Samuel Coleridge and Thomas de Quincey were beginning their addictive commitments to opium (also called laudanum). The addiction of many writers of the romantic period to opiate drugs derives from the capacity of those chemicals to induce dreamlike states of consciousness. These transcendent states often occur during sleep, and they sometimes occur immediately upon closing the eyes at sleep onset. Rarely, they even invade waking. Coleridge used his drug experience to inspire the immortal Kubla Khan verses, and de Quincey left us a remarkable account of his own experience with opium.

De Quincey's account lends itself well to analysis using the knowledge gained through modern sleep and dream pharmacology. It helps us to answer the question: What is the mechanism of action of the opiates upon the brain and how might it intensify dreaming?

Thomas de Quincey: The Fierce Chemistry of Dreams

In his famous *Confessions of an English Opium Eater* De Quincey (figure 14.1) is very clear on three important points. First, between 1804 and 1812 (when he used opium on a disciplined and regularly intermittent twice weekly basis), he experienced no symptoms of intoxication, no disturbances of intellectual function, and no striking alterations of consciousness. Second, even after 1814 (when he became a daily user), he experienced nothing but relief of the depression that had afflicted him since 1813, and he could still read and study with good concentration and pleasure. Finally, by 1816 (when he was so thoroughly addicted that he could no longer focus attention on his work), he was regularly beset by intensely unpleasant dreams and by sleep onset visions that sound very much like hypnagogic hallucinations.

These visions, which de Quincey ascribed to "the reawakening of a *state of the eye* generally incident to childhood, or *exalted states of irritability*," were distressing in part because they were involuntary. As a child once said to him, "I can tell them to go, and they go; but sometimes they come when I don't tell them to come."

Here is his own vivid description of these dreamlike experiences.

In the middle of 1817, I think it was, this faculty became positively distressing to me: at night, when I lay awake in bed, vast processions passed along in mournful pomp; friezes of never-ending stories, that to my feelings were as sad and solemn as if they were stories drawn from times before Oedipus or Priam before Tyre—before Memphis. And, at the same time, a corresponding change took place in my dreams; a theatre seemed suddenly opened and *lighted up within my brain*, which presented nightly spectacles of more than earthly splendour. (*Confessions*, p. 60; italics mine)

The link between these unbidden hypnagogic images and nocturnal dreaming was apparent to de Quincey, and he astutely inferred that both were due to an increase in the excitability of his visual brain:

As the creative state of the eye increased, a sympathy seemed to arise between the waking and the dreaming states of the brain in one point—that whatsoever I happened to call up and to trace by a voluntary act upon the darkness was very apt to transfer itself to my dreams; so that I feared to exercise this faculty; for, as Midas turned all things to gold, that yet baffled his hopes and defrauded his human desires, so whatsoever things capable of being visually represented I did but think of in the darkness, immediately shaped themselves into phantoms of the eye; and, by a process apparently no less inevitable, when thus once traced in faint and visionary colours, like writings in sympathetic ink, they were drawn out by the fierce chemistry of my dreams, into insufferable splendour that fretted my heart. (*Confessions*, p. 60)

De Quincey thus discovered that via the "fierce chemistry" of dreams he could immediately translate thoughts into visual images, but that the price of this artifice was negative emotion! "For this, and all other

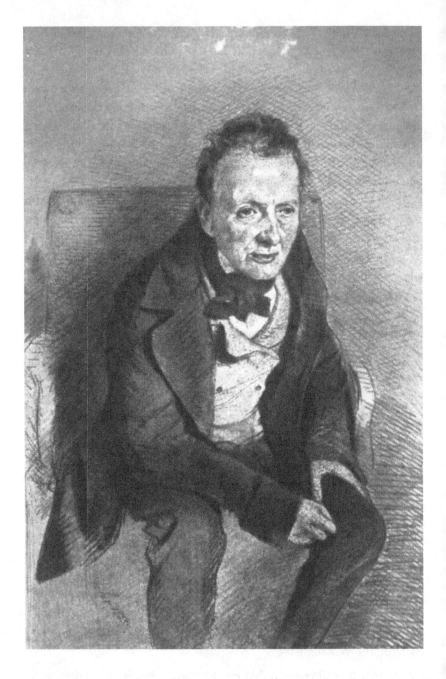

changes in my dreams, were accompanied by deep-seated anxiety and gloomy melancholy, such as are wholly incommunicable by words" (*Confessions,* p. 60).

It seems reasonable to propose that de Quincey's brain had been altered by its long exposure to opiates. What could that alteration be and by what mechanism could it intensify dreaming to this intolerable psyche-delic extent? Before attempting to answer these questions, let us note two other points that de Quincey emphasized regarding the formal qualities of dreams. In addition to visual hallucinosis and emotional intensifica-tion, he noted marked alterations in orientation and memory, two aspects of cognition that are disrupted in normal dreaming. Orientation was al-tered as follows:

Buildings, landscapes, &c. were exhibited in proportions so vast as the bodily eye is not fitted to receive. Space swelled, and was amplified to an extent of unut-terable infinity. This, however, did not disturb me so much as the vast expansion of time; I sometimes seemed to have lived for 70 or 100 years in one night; nay, sometimes had feelings representative of a millennium passed in that time, or, however, of a duration far beyond the limits of any human experience. (*Confes-sions,* p. 61)

This does not appear to be simply an exaggeration of normal dream dis-orientation, but it certainly does resemble some descriptions of psyche-delic drug states. Likewise, the memory enhancement that is typical of normal dreaming is massively exceeded in what sounds for all the world like the description of false memories that subjects in hypnotic trance states often give:

The minutest incidents of childhood, or forgotten scenes of later years, were often revived: I could not be said to recollect them; for if I had been told of them when waking, I should not have been able to acknowledge them as parts of my past

---

Figure 14.1
The author of *Confessions of an English Opium Eater,* Thomas de Quincey (1785–1859) was an idealistic romantic who abandoned his early poetic ambi-tions, hoping to become the intellectual benefactor of mankind by being "the first founder of a true philosophy." His central idea, that pain and grief were essential to the development of the soul, was vividly enacted in his vagabond life. His use of opium cost him any possibility of a stable social or work life, but he tried to turn this adversity to advantage by describing his "dreams and noonday visions" as the "crowning grace" of his life work. (From Edmund Gosse, *Outline of Litera-ture,* vol. 4, 1904)

experience. But placed as they were before me, in dreams like intuitions, and clothed in all their evanescent circumstances and accompanying feelings, *I recognised* them instantaneously. (*Confessions*, p. 61)

We can understand the collaboration of long years of opium abuse with the autocreativity of the dreaming brain via an analysis of the indeed fierce chemistry of dreams that de Quincey could only poetically imagine.

The opiates give their initially pleasurable effects by occupying the receptors of those aminergic brainstem neurons that enhance waking. By overactivating those cells they confer euphoria by energizing the brain. This was the response that de Quincey sought—and found— in the first phase of his opium eating life. Because his use was intermittent, he was able to appreciate these stimulant effects over and over again without compromising his cognitive capacities. But when, in phase II, he tried to treat the depression that may have been precipitated by his phase I bingeing, his temporary success was converted, via the habituation of constant dosing, to an addiction that, in phase III, became a pharmacologically sustained state of delirium that was ultimately more disabling than the depression it was designed to correct.

As the aminergic system of his brain became habituated, de Quincey was obliged to take excessive amounts of opium to stave off a withdrawal reaction, and, as in the case of alcohol abuse, he was brought to the edge of delirium by the tendency of his long-suppressed REM sleep generation mechanisms to escape from opiate inhibition. The suppression of REM occurs in part because the aminergic system that opium enhances inhibits REM. In phase I, this suppression was only acute and hence easily and rapidly compensated. In phase II, physiological recovery became more and more difficult, and by the time de Quincey entered phase III, it was impossible. This is because the cholinergic system was progressively gaining more and more force, mediating an enhancement of REM that was so strong as to break through into waking (the hypnagogic imagery), to greatly exaggerate and distort dreaming, and to evoke profoundly unpleasant feelings.

The ultimate irony, of course, is that in the end de Quincey was suffering not only from delirium, but also from an opiate-induced depression. Not only had he altered his waking and dream consciousness through his opium abuse, but he had also driven his affective system into a corner from which there was no escape. When de Quincey died in 1859, he was a solitary and eccentric inhabitant of the opium dreams he immortalized in his *Confessions*.

All of the opium freaks of the early nineteenth century were obligated to eat their opium, which was both a curse (because they needed huge quantities to compensate for the impurity and because the gastrointestinal side effects were prominent) and a blessing (because they were spared the likelihood of fatal overdosing, infections, and pulmonary emboli that followed the invention of the hypodermic syringe by Alex Wood in 1853). By injecting pure morphine, the acute euphoria, the famous rush, and the relief of the addiction-related craving were all enhanced because more of the drug could reach the brain more quickly. When heroin was synthesized by adding two acetyl groups to the morphine molecule, entry into the brain was further favored over absorption into body fat of the pleasure giving, pain killing molecules.

When morphine enters the brain, where does it go? And could its possibly preferential binding by the neuronal receptors of specific brain regions help us understand its effects on the subjective experience of pain, of pleasure, and of dreams? Obtaining answers to these questions became possible in the 1970s, thanks to the work of Michael Kuhar, Solomon Snyder, and Candace Pert at the Johns Hopkins University School of Medicine. By developing methods for identifying specific receptors in microscopic brain sections (Kuhar) and simultaneously measuring the quantitative binding affinity of various compounds in vitro (Pert and Snyder), the Hopkins group was able to deduce the most likely sites of opiate action in the brain (table 14.1).

When the opiates occupy receptors that normally mediate pain and pain is mollified, the hypothesis is that either the transmission of pain impulses or the neuronal circuits involved in their perception are blocked. The neuronal interpretation is supported by many subjects' claims that they could still feel the pain but that it no longer bothered them. I remember seeing the Boston Theater Company production of Bertholt Brecht's *Galileo* shortly after having two deeply impacted wisdom teeth chiseled out of my jaw by a dental surgeon. In addition to feeling the two huge holes in my mouth, I was aware of deep throbbing pain, but I had no

Table 14.1
Opiate Receptors and Subjective Experience

Subjective Phenomenon	Receptors Labeled
Pain	
Body	Spinal cord laminal I & II
Head	Substantia gelatinosa
Perception	Thalamic nuclei
Euphoria	Locus coeruleus
	Parabrachial nucleus
Emotion	Amygdala
	Stria terminalis
	Habenula and interpeduncular nuclei
	Fasciculus retroflexus

difficulty attending to and even enjoying the play. In fact, I chuckled to myself throughout and occasionally even burst out laughing, although as anyone who has seen *Galileo* knows, it is not a comedy and contains no jokes! So what was going on?

Sixty milligrams of codeine is what was going on. These morphine-like molecules were coating my thalamic pain perception relay neurons, making my jaw pain seem almost incidental. Were my euphoria and fatuous giggling caused by the molecular goosing of my locus coeruleus, my interpendicular nucleus, and my amygdala? Surely, these systems should not be activated by having their receptors occupied by a block-ade of neurotransmission. No, it seems more likely that my silly giddi-ness was a release phenomenon caused by the disinhibition of other emotion systems of the brain that are normally restrained by noradre-nergic inhibition or counterbalanced by amygdala-mediating negative emotions.

The plausibility of this hypothesis is supported, in part, by the psycho-physiology of dreaming, which, as we began this chapter by pointing out, is both analgesic and hyperemotional. But instead of blocking the tha-lamic and locus coeruleus opiate receptors, REM sleep simply shuts down the locus coeruleus (norepinephrine) and the raphé (serotonin) systems, so that many parts of the brain are disinhibited. Is dreaming euphoric? Not always. In fact, the leading emotion is anxiety. But elation (euphoria) is in second place, and many of my dreams are as incongruously comical

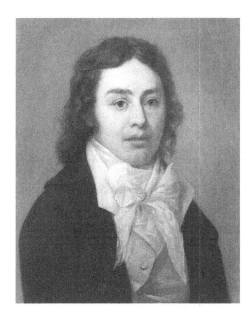

Figure 14.2
The co-creator, with William Wordsworth, of the "Lyrical Ballads" was Samuel
Coleridge (1772–1834), who is of great interest to the themes of the Dream Drugstore for two important reasons. The first is that his famous Kubla Khan poem
is thought to be the product of an opium dream. In any case Coleridge, like de
Quincey, was both seriously addicted to opium and had a falling out with Wordsworth. The second is that he was so greatly influenced by David Hartley, the
founder of associationist psychology, that he named his son Hartley, and tried
for a time to understand the mind, including dreams, scientifically. Impatient with
science, he turned to transcendentalism. (Courtesy of the National Portrait Gallery, London)

as my bizarre response to Brecht's *Galileo*. So why don't I take codeine
more often? One answer is that I don't have to have my wisdom teeth
extracted more than once; another is that I am afraid of addiction. But
the best answer is that I have a highly reliable, safe, and potent way of
achieving the psychedelic effects that the drugs enhance. I just go to bed,
sleep, and dream. The drugstore in my brain does the rest. One dream
prescription, filled by my cerebral pharmacist, is presented here to illustrate the power of autosuggestion in the creation of dream architecture
every bit as fabulous as those described by the drug-using poets (figure
14.2).

Caverns Measureless to Man: A Naturalistic Reply to Samuel Coleridge and Thomas de Quincey

5/10/99 Monday

I awakened in the early morning with recall of a wild racing, flying, falling dream that was one of my longest and most complex dreams ever. The dream occurred in recovery sleep following a weekend outing to Rowley, Newburyport, and Plum Island, where I had not slept well because our family of five, including our rambunctious three-year-old twins, was lodged in a single attic loft. On the Saturday morning of our departure I found a copy of Thomas de Quincey's *Confessions of an Opium Eater* in the Brookline bookstore, some passages of which I had already been given by my colleague Hellmut Wohl, and I took it along to read. I mention all these points to suggest that my own exotic dream was possibly prompted by REM deprivation and primed by the text of Thomas de Quincey. It certainly had nothing to do with exogenous drugs.

I was on a racing bicycle. Like my old Kestrel, the dream bike was very lightweight and fast, but also flimsy and unstable. I was whizzing along when I realized I was going the wrong way (perhaps to Colorado?). To correct my direction, I made a daring and hazardous U-turn, followed by a series of dizzying swerves to avoid oncoming cars.

I entered a cave in the deep mountains where it seemed that I was to meet Steve Foote. Steve was busy (giving a talk), and I supposed that I could save time by making a shortcut through the cave. I plunged ahead, but by now I was afoot and/or even flying, although it still felt like an extension of my bike ride. I remember thinking "it shouldn't take me more than a day to get to Colorado" (or was it back to Boston?).

My flying was hampered by the uneven, jagged, and steep walls of the cave, which was structured like an immense gallery with a helical twisting course in its upper reaches. I was having the usual mix of conviction (of course I can fly!) and doubt (flying is impossible!), and the associated emotions of elation and fear.

By the way, the cave had some manmade aspects—like reinforced concrete supports in the walls—and it was as architecturally grandiose as it was gothic and forbidding. I found all of this a bit strange, but not strange enough to make me suspect that I was dreaming.

As I neared the top of the cave, where I could see light but no egress, I seemed to be held aloft by a harness connected to what might have been wings, and I felt uneasy about this. I said to myself, "You are 65, and the father of two three-year-olds, much too old and with too many responsibilities to be flying around in a cave." This reasonable reservation was quickly swept away by the resumption of my vertiginous flight.

I navigated out of the high pocket in the top of the cave that I had mistaken for an exit and found myself 200–300 feet up in the main cavern. All of a sudden I began to plunge downward. This was unpleasant, as I imagined crashing, but I was able to reassure myself that, after all, I obviously *could* fly because I had gotten up that high under my own steam! And my landing was, happily, soft.

But now I had to confront Steve and explain to him why I had come back but couldn't stay. I had to get back to Boston. But whether I set off or not—or simply woke up—I can't remember. But I *did* wake up, and noticed that it was 4:00 A.M. In order to fix such recall as I now report, I lay still and reflected upon my awesome experience.

I am not suggesting either that my cavern dream can match de Quincey's architectural extravaganza or that my account of it is in the same league as Coleridge's Kubla Khan. Dreaming, psychedelic drug states, and artistic creation are *not* identical. But they are analogous. Many dreams possess just those qualities drug users seek, and by public waking standards, *all* dreams are autocreative and, if not artistic, they are as gloriously fabulous to the dreamer as any painting, film, or poem.

But the real payoff of exotic dreaming is its naturalism. By virtue of being a product of apparently life-sustaining brain activation in sleep, it is not only necessary but free of charge, free of assault trauma, and free of long-term health risks.

15

From Cult to Laboratory: Mushrooms, Cactus Buttons, and Coca Leaves

Recreational drug taking is almost always a response to the human yearning for transcendence. And dreaming, too, can be a vehicle to never-never land. Thus drug and dream cults can arise as easily in modern day California as they did in pre-Columbian Mexico. Altered states of consciousness with high degrees of instability, plasticity, and—above all—hallucinatory proclivity are of obvious utility to those seeking to establish themselves as prophets, priests, seers, shamans, or gurus, and to their would-be disciples.

Many cultures have discovered plants with the power to potentiate visual illusions and/or hallucinations, and used them in religious or tribal rituals. In some cases we know the molecular structure of the active ingredients, and in all of these cases the similarity to the brain molecules that impede or release dreaming is striking.

Two good examples are the peyote cactus (which contains mescaline) and the magic mushroom (which contains psilocybin). Both were discovered and used by the Mexican Indians and both have been so thoroughly analyzed biochemically that their active ingredients have been synthesized.

The intervention of science in the synthesis of these potent molecules does no more to quell the cult use of the drugs than the neurophysiology of sleep dampens the ardor of dream cult adherents! People just can't accept the limitations of the scientific world view. Even if it is reckless, groundless, or dangerous to health, they want to go beyond common sense, to defy gravity, or obtain communion with the beyond.

Peyote, Mescaline, and Its Synthetic Relatives

In the case of peyote, whose effects Heinrich Klüver described so thoroughly and Aldous Huxley later made famous in *The Doors of Perception,* the route to chemical synthesis did not stop at mescaline (which was identified by Haffer and synthesized by Spaets in 1918). Because it was so weak and so upsetting to the subject's gastrointestinal tract, Alexander Shulgin modified the molecule in the 1960s, resulting in a whole family of popular street drugs that are still making the rounds of the U.S. underground. These include TMA, the amphetamine derivatives of mescaline, MDMA (Ecstasy), DOET, and DOM (see figure 12.1). As with the amphetamines themselves, these agents could (in low doses) enhance self-awareness and euphoria and produce visual distortions or hallucinations, or (in higher doses) blow the top off the mind. The increased potency of these synthetic drugs was due to the addition of the methyl group, which impedes enzymatic attack on the molecules. In fact, DOM's popularity among the California hippies was due to its extremely long-lasting action. They called it STP, for serenity, tranquillity, and peace. As far as our story is concerned, all of these molecules are mimics of the amine modulators that inhibit sleep and REM.

The Psilocybe Mushroom and Psilocybin

The use of psychoactive mushrooms in Central America dates back to before 500 B.C., when Mexican Indians called them *teonanactl,* or Food of the Gods, because they were thought to carry prophetic messages from the deity, just as dreams were seen as prophecies from pre-Biblical times to the present.

The great botanist Richard Schultes and the biochemist Albert Hofmann (of LSD fame) celebrated the wide variety of organisms with these properties in a book called *Plants of the Gods.* When I first met Schultes, in summer of 1986 at the Rockefeller Study Center in Bellagio, Italy, he told me that although he had enjoyed the psychedelic effects of many plants, he had never recalled a single natural dream!

Gordon and Valentine Wasson made the discovery of the psilocybe mushroom, from which Hofmann later isolated psilocin and psilocybin.

They obtained the teonanactl plant from Mexicans whose trust they had won over enough to allow them to participate in a sacred mushroom ceremony. Roger Herr identified the teonanactl mushroom as *Psilocybe Mexicana,* and he asked Hofmann to do the biochemical analysis. Unable to establish a bioassay for the extracts he made from the mushrooms, Hofmann took the psilocin and psilocybin extracts himself and reported vivid subjective experiences that were similar to those of LSD. LSD, psilocin, and psilocybin were all similar to serotonin in their molecular structure.

Heinrich Klüver, Mescaline, and the Temporal Lobe

What do the vision inducing effects of mescaline and the behavior altering effects of experimental damage to the temporal lobe have in common? One answer is Heinrich Klüver, the scientist who first described both of these apparently unrelated phenomena in detail. A more profound answer is that taken together the two phenomena demonstrate the importance of molecular and brain structure in shaping mind and behavior. Beyond that, we now have good reason to suppose that the temporal lobe might mediate some of the more extreme effects of mescaline. This mechanism was unsuspected by Klüver, but his work helped set the stage for it.

Mescaline is a molecule whose chemical structure is analogous to the natural neurotransmitters epinephrine, norepinephrine, and dopamine, and it most likely exerts its psychedelic effects by interfering with the normal modulation of perception that permits us to see without hallucinating (see again figure 12.1). In dreaming, we hallucinate without actually seeing because neuromodulators like norepinephrine are not available, a situation akin to mescaline psychosis. The German biochemist E. Spaeth first worked out the chemical structure of mescaline in 1918, following up on its identification as an active constituent of peyote, the cactus buttons that Mexican Indian shamans have used for centuries to induce visions as part of their religious practices.

As we learned in chapter 9, the temporal lobe is a deep forebrain structure that is particularly prone to seizures; these seizures may induce dreaminess and hyperreligiosity. These traits have been noted by many medical authorities and were celebrated by the writer Fyodor Dostoyevsky in his novels *The Idiot* and *The Brothers Karamazov.* Dostoyevsky spoke authoritatively because he himself suffered from temporal lobe epilepsy. In the more recent annals of modern brain science, no story is perhaps better known than the evocation of dreamlike recollections and sensations in epileptic patients whose temporal lobes were electrically stimulated by the Canadian neurosurgeon Wilder Penfield. Now that we know that temporal lobe activation is a normal aspect of REM sleep, we begin to see how all of these diverse strands can come together.

Heinrich Klüver, who devoted his scientific career to understanding the brain mechanisms of perception, was naturally fascinated by the experimental possibility of chemically altering perception (figure 15.1). Born in 1897, he was 21 when mescaline first became available and 23 when he himself first took the drug. Within ten years he had conducted and published the first systematic study of its effects (*Mescal and Mechanisms of Hallucinations,* 1928).

Klüver's classic work first reviews the history of mescaline's effect on the visual system and then proposes a general theory of visual hallucination that focuses sharply on the analogy between mescaline visions and dreaming. Klüver recognized that the occurrence of visual hallucinations in dreams strongly favored a central brain component in their genesis, an idea that was then quite novel because all visual perception was thought to be dependent on the retina. The persistence of visual dreams in people whose retinae have been damaged now prove Klüver's point. Here is a capital passage from Klüver's book:

At this point, attention should be called to certain facts that may prove to be of interest in connection with physiological or psychological studies of dreams. Since, in most dreams, visual elements are dominant and since striking alterations in the visual sphere are characteristic of mescaline effects, it seems reasonable to expect an enhancement of dream phenomena under the influence of mescaline. An analysis of available data, however, indicates that most subjects report an absence of dreams for the night following the intoxication, and others refer only to "ordinary dreams." Even though the night may have been dreamless, the next day often provides evidence that the visual system has not yet returned to its normal state. In the literature, the author found only one reference to "unusually plastic, colorful dreams," the nature of which was not described. It seems, therefore, that contrary to our expectations, mescaline does not lead to an enhancement of dreams and that it may even suppress dream activity. This can be only a tentative conclusion, since the whole problem has not been systematically investigated. We know nothing about the effects in chronic mescalinism. (p. 86)

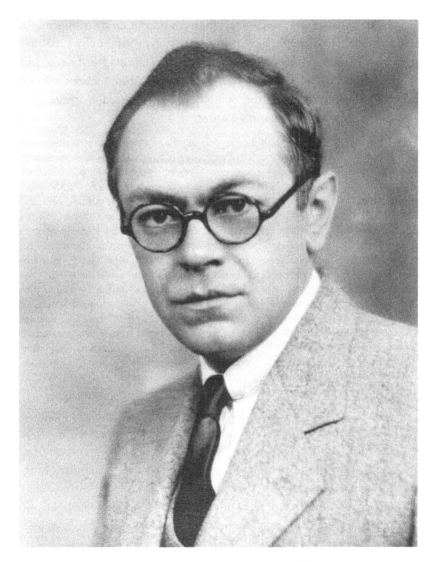

Figure 15.1
Heinrich Klüver (1897–1979) was Albert Hofmann's equal in detailed self-description, but his altered states of consciousness were no accident. Because he was an experimental psychologist who was interested in eidetic imagery (popularly known as photographic memory), he used mescaline to induce hallucinations in humans, including himself, with a view to understanding their cerebral basis through experiments in animals. His descriptions of mescaline's effects, which are quoted extensively in the text, keenly note similarities with dreaming long before there was any suspicion of a mechanistic analogy between the natural and drug-induced states. (Reprinted with permission from the University of Chicago Library)

We can now explain the counterintuitive notion that mescaline might suppress normal dreaming by recognizing that many of the chemical analogues of the modulators of waking perception suppress REM sleep, and with it nocturnal dreams. It is only as the effects of mescaline are declining and REM sleep is escaping from inhibition that psychedelic dreams, like this one reported by Klüver, may occur:

> I am lying in bed in a large hall. It seems to me that there are many similar beds in this hall which are also occupied. I turn over to my right side and see a large window which I subject to close inspection. I see clearly the following black letters R E S T A U R. It surprises me that I can even distinguish letters. To the right of the last R is a vertical pipe, and I am aware of the fact that it covers additional letters. In the window is a large bottle containing red liquid. There are three words on this bottle. These words are complete and meaningful; yet I am dissatisfied with the third word, because I feel that it is somehow too short. The words are surrounded by a reticulated pattern in delicate greenish colors giving the effect of a decorative label. The scene suddenly shifts, and I find myself looking at the gray wall of a house. Very delicate and fragile objects resembling unshelled peanuts are regularly distributed over the whole surface, thus forming a latticelike pattern. Each husk stands on end, forming an angle of approximately 45 degrees with the surface of the wall. Violet clouds pass across the surface. This makes me wonder whether the whole phenomenon is merely a hallucination. To determine whether such is the case I close my eyes; but I still see violet clouds. I conclude that the house and the peanut lattice have objective existence and that the violet clouds are of hallucinatory origin. (pp. 87–88)

Klüver acknowledged that mescaline probably influenced the retina as well as the visual brain because it first produced effects that he called visual "form constants," such as gratings, lattices, and fretworks, betokening activation of neurons in the early stages of visual processing. John Dowling has shown that dopamine plays a key role in the physiology of the retinal ganglia cells that convert the photon energy of light into neural signals that come to represent edges and bars once they have been processed by the lateral geniculate body of the thalamus. The geniculate is the first point at which the central neuromodulators norepinephrine and serotonin that are involved in dream generation can interact with signals of retinal origin.

Following ingestion of mescaline, one first sees spirals, tunnels, funnels, and alleys. Then scenes picturing episodes become connected much as they do in dreams. One sees this very same progression, from geometric forms, through synesthesia, to architectural visions, at sleep onset when the visual system is shifting its attention away from external stimuli to more internal ones. Furthermore, entopic phenomena like phosgenes and hypnagogic hallucinations are common to both natural dreaming and mescal-induced states. At very high doses of mescaline, frank psychosis may emerge; expressive faces, time distortions, discontinuity of image, and active and intense emotions then predominate.

The emotions mescaline evokes are not always pleasant. Although one may feel euphoria and a sense of cosmic transcendence, one may also see grotesque faces and have a gripping sense of terror. By this time, the brain effects have spread far beyond the visual system. More specifically, they have by now clearly engaged those limbic structures that constituted Klüver's second scientific focus of interest.

Working with his colleague Paul Bucy at the University of Chicago (where by 1933 he had become a professor), Klüver showed that damage to the structures of the temporal lobe of monkeys produced, first, a release of exploratory behavior most strikingly seen as a tendency to lick and sniff indiscriminately and a propensity to put whatever object was available into the mouth. At the same time, previously aggressive monkeys became very fearful and docile. This "taming" effect is the second element in the Klüver-Bucy syndrome, whose description constitutes a landmark in the history of limbic lobe neuroscience. Klüver and Bucy's findings helped to establish the brain itself as the site of emotional experience. While signals from the body may contribute to our feelings of anxiety or rage, they are not essential, as William James had asserted.

Recent studies of dream emotion prove Klüver and Bucy's point. They support the idea that it is the brain itself—and more specifically the limbic brain—that may generate fear (the number one dream affect), cosmic elation (number two), and anger (number three). To round out the picture, there are reports that an intensification of these same emotions colors the dreams of patients with temporal lobe epilepsy. Subjects may indeed evince rapid heart action, increases in blood pressure, and rises and falls of breathing efforts in REM sleep, but these are not sensed as part of the subjective experience of dream emotion.

Klüver's emphasis on form constants in his human mescaline work and his formal analysis of emotional behavior in his monkey lesion studies are scientifically exemplary. Although individuals vary widely in exactly what formal elements are present and to what degree they influence dream content, these formal features constitute universals that must be the foundational beginnings of any scientific theory of perception and emotion in psychosis and in dreaming. The work of scientists like Klüver and Hofmann provides an important counterpoint in the descriptive poverty of the cult of psychedelic drug use.

The Cult of Dreaming and Psychedelic Drug Use

What about the cult of dreaming? To what end do dream cultists ride the natural psychedelic wave that rolls ashore when serotinin and norepinephine neurons are turned off and the cholinergic system is unleashed? Like Carlos Casteneda, they like to fly, and like aphrodisiac addicts they like to make love. Without the risk of drug hangover, many dreamers succeed in attaining these elevating, hedonistic effects. Few are as ambitious as Emmanuel Swedenborg, who summoned dream angels and received instructions from them about the foundation of the Church of the New Jerusalem, or William Blake, whose oneiric tutor taught him what to paint and how to paint it.

Many of the letters that I receive report, with firm conviction, that dreams can predict the future, make clear the meaning of the past, explain the workings of the universe, and reveal the intentions of God, and even provide communicative channels to the afterlife! One might come to the conclusion that REM sleep is the physiological basis of religion! All these claims have been made by psychedelic drug exponents, too. And some of them have even advocated psychedelic drug use to enhance dreaming, all in the service of enlightenment.

William James was wise to insist that we should be open to such claims, to hear them out, and to weigh them critically in developing our models of the mind. To be rational, logical, and analytical may be a good way to find things out scientifically. To be imaginative, inspired, and believing may be a good way to deal with our ignorance of the many things that science has not yet told us and may never ever reveal. As the poles of our cerebral existence, waking and dreaming certainly constitute a remarkably diversified portfolio of mental and spiritual assets. Armed with these native talents I myself am not tempted by psychosis, by psychedelics, or by spiritualism. It's not just that I don't like losing control, being even slightly mad, or naively gullible. I simply find that I can achieve satisfaction without those props. To help convince you that you don't need to take drugs to have a psychedelic experience, I share the following dream report with you.

A Psychedelic Dream

At first the flower on the table did not seem exceptional, even though it was clearly both alive and artificial. I tried to remember the name of the oriental plant that it resembled. Could it be ginger? I have seen flowers like these in hotels in Maui, Hawaii, in Cancun, Mexico, and even in the Copley Plaza in Boston. They have a distinctive color between red and very hot pink, the leaves are deep green with a waxy sheen, and some of the corolla petals are white.

I was sharing my appreciation of this exotic bloom with my daughter, Julia, who was seated with me at a table on which the flower sat. To our amazement the flower then increased about four times in both size and vividness of coloration. I ascribed this metamorphosis to the process by which Chinese paper flowers rapidly bloom when placed in water. The paper simply expands as it absorbs the moisture and dyes in the paper give it a more intense color as they go into solution.

This horticultural extravaganza immediately followed an ecstatic run downhill on skis. I explained to my old friend and crony, Peter Thompson, that my first run was so painfully awkward that I was hesitant to try again. But, as is often the case, I found my ski legs on the second run and I swerved, cut, jumped, and carved my way rapidly downhill through the soft spring snow. Peter said that he had not tried to ski in years but remembered our early adventures on the slopes together and asked me to take him with me again. I said, "Sure."

When I got up from the flower table I realized that I was a bit lost. Where were these strange events taking place? When I checked my left back pocket for my wallet (as I always do when I get up to move), I was startled to find that it was missing. The anxiety, which is normally completely quelled by my finding the wallet in place, augmented radically. But when I realized that the wallet was safely ensconced in my *right* back pocket (where I *never* put it), my anxiety immediately subsided. I was then able to find my way out of the maze-like fence enclosure that had me quite buffaloed for a moment or two.

When I awakened it was 6:58 A.M., and the room was flooded with spring light. I could hear my twin sons, Andrew and Matthew, chatting in the next room. My head was heavy with sleep and I wanted to go back to the dream world, but by the time I had gone to the bathroom and peeked out at the daffodils blooming in my garden, I decided to get up. While brushing my teeth and proffering prepared tooth brushes to my two three-year-olds, it was only by dint of extreme mental effort I was able to rescue these three dream fragments from the ashbin of amnesia.

Why am I sleeping so heavily, I wondered? The clocks had sprung forward by an hour just two days ago in honor of the vernal equinox, so we all had a mild case of jet lag that morning. And after gardening avidly on both days of the Easter weekend, I had biked five miles on my way home from work. But still, this sleep was unusually hard to shake and these exotic dreams unusually difficult to recall.

I didn't realize until later that morning that they graphically illustrated my response to Aldous Huxley's *Heaven and Hell,* that slim and distressingly slight volume that I read just before my bike ride home the day before. For Huxley, Heaven represents the ecstasy of psychedelic experience, whereas Hell is the agony of psychosis. Huxley recognized that both the ecstasy and the agony are primed by chemical changes in the brain, but he was convinced that the cerebral valve was simply a portal for influences from the beyond. For Huxley, the brain mechanisms were necessary but not sufficient to account for those perceptual transports. That's why he called them visions (if they had a heavenly origin) or hallucinations (if they had a hellish one).

One reason for Huxley's denial of the adequacy of brain mechanisms in accounting for such imagery may be the very same kind of poor dream recall that hindered my recollection of the flower, the ski run, and the maze. Huxley was agreeing with Calvin Hall when he said, "Only one dream in three is colored, or has some color in it." If Huxley had tried harder to overcome his poor dream recall he would have realized that intense, "preternaturally brilliant" color was not the unique hallmark of visions induced by drugs like mescaline or by practices like hypnosis or meditation.

Although I did not consciously incubate the gloriously colorful ginger flower of this morning's dream, it clearly and directly counters not only Huxley and Hall, but also all others who fail to recognize that it is the generally poor memory for dreams that leads to the belief that they are typically colorless. The fact that dream visions can be as vividly colorful and as metaphoric as my rapidly expanding ginger flower clearly indicates that there is no qualitative difference between dreaming and psychedelic visionary perception.

Unless one retains the medieval view that even dreaming is caused by some vagabond genie from the spirit world (who squeezes through the cerebral valve in sleep), the most parsimonious (and, to me, completely adequate) hypothesis is that dreams, psychedelic and hypnotic visions, and psychosis are all caused by functional changes in the brain.

Intellectual parsimony is not the only economy of the altered brain function hypothesis. Whether or not psychedelic dreams are as pleasurable and as fascinating as artificial and pathological visions, they also have numerous advantages to recommend them: they are ludicrously inexpensive (because they are free); they are nontoxic (because no exogenous chemical need be ingested); they are methodologically simple (because no other person need be hired or conscripted); they are safe (because no outward behavior is associated with them); and they can be abruptly terminated (simply by waking up). And, as far as we know, there are no cumulative or delayed side effects of dreaming.

Of course, there is no guarantee that all dreams will be ecstatic. In point of fact, they are considerably more likely to be hellish than heavenly. A temporarily lost wallet is not the most diabolical experience I have had in dreams. Deadly force is worse (as in those thankfully rare attacks by dream dive-bombers), but anxious uncertainty about who, what, when, and where is the rule and it sometimes rises to—and remains at—panic level.

So dreaming can be a good trip (ecstatic elation as in my second ski run is not uncommon) or a bad trip (with negative emotions like anxiety, fear, and anger always popping up). This means that dreaming is *both* heaven and hell (or that heaven and hell are virtual realities that are fabricated by us to mirror the virtual reality of our dream experiences). This reversal of Huxley's mystical reading of ecstatic visions is paralleled by the monistic notion that all of the states of interest are not only exclusively cerebral but that they are all caused by common properties of the cerebrum, those chemical control systems of the brain stem that determine natural sequences of conscious states.

Huxley comes closest to this viewpoint when he recognizes the multiple physical predispositions to visionary experience that account for its much greater frequency in the early history of Western culture. When a would-be communicant wanted to get in touch with the other world, a manual of deprivation techniques was at hand: isolation from society (which characterized the hermetic retreat); fasting (which was encouraged during the most holy days); sleep deprivation vigil (which was associated with incantational ritual); dancing, walking, or even whipping (which inflicted physical stress on the supplicant); singing and chanting (which induced hypnoid trance); and powerful suggestion (which was supplied by priests and shamans).

I myself have made the whole trip with sleep deprivation alone. Visitors from the beyond have invaded my sleep lab as I sat entranced by the buzzing pens of the polygraph. Menacing strangers have invaded my woodshed as I stacked kindling after an all-night vigil on an airplane headed east from California. And imaginary co-pilots have encouraged me to stay awake as I drove late at night in the penumbra of highway hypnosis.

In my case, none of these uninvited image people promised salvation. They didn't even reveal scientific secrets. But they did, by their presence, make one thing clear: that sleep deprivation alone can open wide the Doors of Perception that Huxley celebrated. Had I prepared my mind for specific communications from the beyond, I have no doubt that my visionary visitors would have articulated whatever words I wanted to hear. The point is that you don't need a drug, you don't need a medium, and you certainly don't need a spirit world to have them. Those exotic ginger flowers and that tumultuous ski run spoke so clearly to the shade of Aldous Huxley: "You are wrong about dreams. They can be both preternaturally colorful and ecstatically animated." Even without mescaline or LSD, and certainly without cocaine, a drug that will almost certainly counteract psychedelic dreaming.

Sigmund Freud's Favorite Drug

One sure way to impede dreaming is to increase the strength of the aminergic modulators like norepinephrine. One can do this by taking the drugs cocaine and amphetamine, which cause an increased release of the natural neuromodulators from pre-synaptic terminals and/or block reuptake with the same net effect. Two of the most legitimate uses of these drugs are the treatment of attention deficit disorder (ADD) and the treatment of narcolepsy. In both conditions the drugs effect an increase in vigilance, where vigilance is defined as the ability to sustain attention to locate a relevant stimulus in a series of irrelevant ones.

The reason that these drugs impede dreaming is that norepinephrine, one of the aminergic neuromodulators that they potentiate, normally promotes waking (and its substate vigilance) and actively inhibits sleep, especially REM sleep. For REM sleep to occur, the norepinephrine system of the locus coeruleus must shut down, in the same way and to the same degree as the serotonin system of the raphé. To the extent that a norepinephrine releasing drug acts in the brain, the chemical balance tips toward waking and away from sleep.

The reason that the illicit use of these drugs is so difficult to curb is not only because they elevate vigilance, but also because they greatly enhance mental energy, elevate mood, increase physical strength, and maximize sexual potency. This sounds like a dream, in the metaphorical sense, and indeed, some actual dreams have these desirable qualities, but the stimulants do not produce otherwise dreamlike mentation even when they trigger psychoses. The similarities between dopamine and cocaine can be appreciated in figure 15.2.

Apropos of cocaine, listen to what the great dream interpreter to be, Sigmund Freud, said in a letter to his fiancée, Martha Bernays, about his favorite drug:

"Woe to you my princess when I come. I will kiss you quite red and feed you til you are plump. And if you are forward, you shall see who is the stronger, a gentle girl who doesn't eat enough or a big wild man who has cocaine in his body" (cited in S. H. Snyder, *Drugs and the Brain*. Scientific American Library 1986, p. 126).

A big wild man, indeed! Freud, the neurasthenic, Freud, the hypochondriac, Freud the somatizing wimp has been transformed by a single

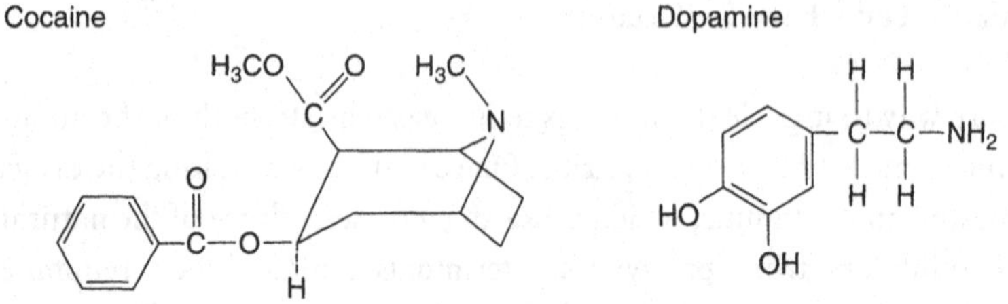

Cocaine

Dopamine

Figure 15.2
Cocaine and dopamine. Cocaine and dopamine both induce a welcome mood enhancement and euphoria as Sigmund Freud and many other users have discovered.

molecule into a tireless sexual acrobat! But in addition to his amorous exploits, Freud also had serious academic ambitions for "coca," which he hoped might counter his patients' nervous exhaustion as it did his own. In his 1884 paper "Uber Coca," Freud said: "I have tested the effect of coca, which wards off hunger, sleep, and fatigue and steels one to intellectual effort, some dozen times in myself."

Notice that the states warded off, hunger, sleep, and fatigue, are all promoters of these restorative, anabolic, energy storing functions that Walter Hess later came to call "trophotropic" (meaning growth enhancing). As Hess correctly surmised, these trophotropic functions are mediated by the cholinergic brain cell systems that are in continuous competitive interaction with the aminergic systems that cocaine boosts. Hess called the energy enhancing effects ergotropic, and, as it turns out, perspicaceously ascribed them to the sympathetic side of the autonomic nervous system. The discovery of the brain cells and molecules that mediate Hess's ergotropic-trophotropic balance system only occurred in the 1960s, at about the same time that street people from Woodstock to Haight-Ashbury were breaking into the Dream Drugstore.

At the cocaine/amphetamine drugstore we thus buy one dream (immediate energy) at the expense of another (long-term restoration). It's a bit like mixed portfolio investing or hedging one's bets. Take a quick hit (and with it, risk) or be patient (and play it safe). As is typical of the ambitious conquistador type, Freud achieved some instant notoriety with his claims for cocaine but incurred doubt about his judgment when the addiction potential that he had underestimated reared its ugly head.

After Freud's prescriptions had hooked his famous colleague and patient Fleishel, the cocaine-induced highs crashed into more and more severe depressions, until Fleishel broke into frank psychosis.

Because cocaine and amphetamine psychoses are anything but psychedelic, they are instructive to examine in terms of our neurobiological hypotheses about why some altered states are dreamlike and others are not. Although cocaine and amphetamines push the dopamine system to the break point, they do not so radically alter the REM sleep modulators, norepinephrine, serotonin, or acetylcholine. Thus, they create a quite different altered state, one more akin to schizophrenia than to dream delirium.

First and foremost, the psychosis does not cloud consciousness in the way that dreaming does. Instead of being disoriented and confused, the stimulant psychotic is clear-headed and knows exactly who and where he or she is, when events are taking place, and what is going on. This lack of what we have called the delirium—like lucid dreaming and some psychotomimetic drug states—is probably due to the fact that the subject's brain-mind is actually being driven away from the REM sleep domain of the AIM state space.

The second major difference is in the nature of the hallucinations and delusions. Instead of being primarily visual as are dream and psychedelic hallucinations, they are more frequently auditory. One hears voices, often accusatory and threatening voices. And instead of being grandiose or fearful confabulations, the delusions are paranoid. Persecution ideas are common. It has always astonished me how rare such delusions are in dreams. Even when there are strong negative emotions like fear and anger, dreamers do not concoct notions of elaborate plots against them. Although there are plenty of villains and heroes in dreams, the FBI, the CIA, and the IRS don't usually figure in.

Snyder suggests that many psychedelic states are like the so-called organic psychoses, whereas the stimulant states are more like the so-called functional psychoses, especially schizophrenia. I agree and add dreaming to the organic category. The schizophrenia analogy is particularly compelling for two reasons: one is because both stimulant psychosis and schizophrenia are remedied by antidopaminergic drugs; the second is that dopamine does not seem to be a player in oneirogenesis.

Why do I use the qualifier "so-called" in this discussion? Because stimulant psychosis—and schizophrenia—must both be as much organic as they are functional. They are just different kinds of organic psychosis from those characterized by delirium. And why are they different? Because the stimulants suppress REM physiology and with it dreaming, whereas the psychedelics enhance REM physiology (or at least some aspects of it).

It is important to recognize that just as waking and REM sleep are two extremes of a continuum, so are the organic and functional factors that contribute to the genesis of psychosis of whatever kind. Even apparently pure psychogenic factors like trauma or abuse must exert their effects on the mind via the brain. How could it be otherwise? It couldn't, and yet our language persists in perpetuating an antique and obsolete mind-brain dualism. The problem is that we don't yet know enough about how ideas and feelings are instantiated in the brain to give an adequate account of the physiological causations associated with them.

Now an obvious question arises. How and why does a stimulant that mimics the aminergic system so as to enhance energy and alertness produce psychosis at all? And why should it produce a schizophrenia-like state? The incomplete and somewhat unsatisfying answer to the first question is that whenever the balance between the aminergic and cholinergic systems is upset—in either direction—psychosis is a likely outcome. When it is hyperaminergic, the psychosis is "functional." When it is hypoaminergic, the psychosis is "organic." The answer to the second question is that auditory hallucinations and paranoid delusions, the features of functional psychosis that stimulants enhance, are actually shared by the affective psychoses (especially mania), as well as by schizophrenia. And mania is even more conspicuously hyperaminergic than schizophrenia!

So it would appear that the brain alertness systems can either be cranked up to a hyperattentive level such that one hears voices and ascribes malevolent intentions to them, or cranked down to so low a level that intrinsic pseudo-sensory signals cause us to see and feel things that we cannot integrate cognitively because our short-term memory capacity is simultaneously disenabled.

Sanity is a delicate balance between the aminergic (ergotropic) and cholinergic (trophotropic) systems of the brain. We normally oscillate safely between two perilous extremes, either of which can be unveiled when we push the system in one direction or the other by introducing chemicals into our bodies. This is one of the main take-home messages from the Dream Drugstore. As if we needed it, this simple but powerful set of rules should help us say no to drugs even when they are offered by a friendly psychiatrist!

Part VI
The Psychological Drugstore

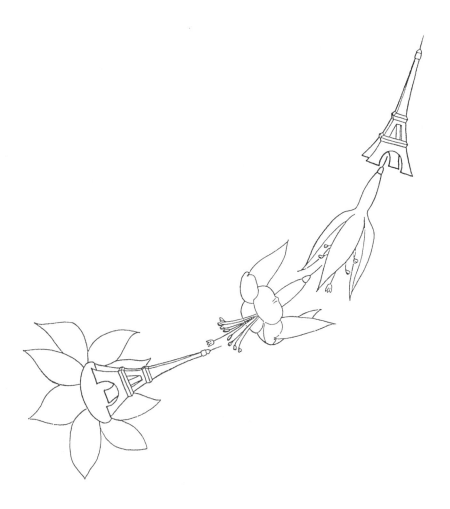

Treatment Implications: Changing the Brain by Changing the Mind

The fields of clinical psychology and clinical psychiatry stand to gain substantial benefits from the principles of the Dream Drugstore. If dreams are caused by chemical mechanisms in the brain, then both our genetic and our personal histories must be encoded there. That is to say, both the form (genetically determined) and the content (experientially determined) of our minds are physically instantiated in our brains and can be read out in the peculiar language of the dream simply by going to sleep. The same brain systems that mediate this mix of genetic and epigenetic information can be tweaked by drugs in the interest of producing altered states of waking with some features of dreams hybridized into them or they can be tempered by medical drugs in the interest of hybridizing some of the features of dreams out of them. To complete our picture, we would like to know how we can alter such a system with purely psychological interventions.

Because modern brain research has stimulated major changes in our way of viewing dreaming and other altered states of consciousness, we have tended to neglect the impact of psychological intervention, and in particular psychotherapy, on self-understanding, improved psychosocial functioning, and more effective behavior. Just as there is no doubt that individual experience determines dream content, there is no doubt that our informed discussion of dreams can be both enlightening and helpful. Besides their didactic power in educating us about the general rules of brain-mind functioning, dreams keep us ever mindful of the reality and impact of emotion in our mental lives.

But how can we bring our knowledge of the brain basis of dream form into psychotherapy? To answer this question, I develop in the first part of this chapter a new set of principles to what I call neurodynamic psychology. I go on to integrate them with guidelines that have stood the test of time in my work as a psychotherapist. The result is a practical code that combines the still valuable residues of the psychoanalytic era with the new brain-based psychology. In the last part of the chapter, I show how psychotherapeutic and other interventions that operate via the mind must simultaneously affect the brain and body. Whether or not conscious experience is itself causal, the brain activity associated with it certainly can be. I can thus change my brain and change my body by changing my mind.

General Principles of Neurodynamic Psychology

The human brain-mind is a complex, dynamic system whose equilibrium depends upon a delicate balancing act between modules within different states of consciousness and whose unity depends upon a well-orchestrated integration across those states. As I have tried to make clear, there are many opportunities for this system to lose equilibrium (balance) and/or to lose unity (integration). These losses are revealed by the close study of normal changes in consciousness across the sleep-waking cycle and a comparison of them to the inadvertent changes that occur in spontaneous psychosis and those that are voluntarily induced by drugs.

One of the most extraordinary, important, and potent features of the brain-mind is the construct of the self. As yet we cannot give an adequate account of how a brain comes to instantiate a self, but this still obscure integration process clearly involves memory and emotion, the two modules of the brain-mind that have always been of greatest interest to psychodynamic psychology. Now that we know how memory and emotion are altered in a state-dependent way, we can use that information to generate new approaches to their access, interpretation, and manipulation in the interest of personal satisfaction and social success.

Before turning to a consideration of how a psychotherapy armed with new knowledge about emotion and memory might proceed, it is crucial to define the position that neurodynamic psychology takes with respect to conscious and unconscious information processing by the brain-mind. I begin with a bottom-up view which assumes that:

1. *Most of the information in the brain-mind is unconscious* and had better remain so. Although it is useful for a neurophysiologist to know

about neurons and neuromodulators, it is not helpful for the average person to think about his or her mind in such terms on a minute-by-minute basis. What is most important for all of us to appreciate is that these fundamental processes are self-organizing and self-regulating. This leads to what could be called the fundamental principle of brain-mind hygiene. Feed it, keep it warm, give it plenty of sleep, and the unconscious brain-mind will usually develop admirably well on its own. The corollary of this deep, vegetative principle is that the brain-mind system itself knows what it wants and needs and signals clearly when its needs are not being met. The astute caregiver—be it parent, therapist, or self—is tuned in to these maintenance signals and responds to them clearly and directly.

2. *Consciousness contains a very small part of the information* in the brain-mind, but it is critical because it is the only channel by which the unconscious can be noticed and voluntarily influenced, and the only portal by which the more complex communications of language can leave or enter the system. Some consider the relatively greater force and size of the unconscious to be an overwhelming adversary to the weak and small conscious mind, but psychoanalysis has greatly exaggerated that view for an initially good reason: to get us to notice the difference. But having accomplished that purpose, psychoanalysis has saddled itself— and us—with a serious error in self-estimation. The top-down side of the neurodynamic model sees consciousness as autonomous in its own special way.

3. *The dynamic relationship of the conscious mind to the unconscious* is the nub of the contrast between the psychoanalytic model and the neurodynamic model. Psychoanalysis sees the unconscious as an enemy constantly needing to be tamed, assuaged, or pacified. Even desire is a primitive impulse that should inspire fear. Human beings are the helpless slaves of sexually possessive, territorially aggressive impulses that well up from the unconscious, constantly threatening maternal incest, patricide, and/or a life of disgraceful compulsions. Unless these impulses are gratified, they are destined to roil around, seeking any lapse in vigilance to escape or to tie themselves and us up in knots of neurotic defense that only cathartic treatment can possibly ameliorate.

4. *Neurodynamics recognizes and respects the power of the unconscious* but is rather more grateful than fearful that so many biologically critical bookkeeping tasks are being taken care of automatically. Rather than viewing the unconscious as an untamable monster with whom only crippling and humiliating compromises can be made, neurodynamic psychology regards it as a sometimes obstreperous mustang that needs to be fenced in, trained, and ridden by a sagacious, patient, and sanguine consciousness cowboy that sees itself as an also gratuitous automatism, but

one particularly blessed by the exceptional powers of evaluation, decision, and voluntary action. Under this umbrella, even happiness is an achievable goal.

5. A key corollary of the shift from the fatalism and inevitability of the psychoanalytic model to the freedom and mutability of neurodynamic psychology is a shift from an emphasis on pathology to an emphasis on health in the view of emotions like anxiety, anger, and desire. Although it is certainly true that any of these emotions can be destructive in excess, it is also true that all of them, in moderation, are adaptive. Neurodynamic psychology can thus claim common ground with a naturalism that is realistically optimistic and an existentialism that helps us live serenely with our complexity.

I fully realize that all of these points are highly debatable and very much in need of more detailed elaboration. My point here is to begin the process of reconceptualizing psychology by laying out a foundational agenda and, at the same time, offering a helping hand to other clinicians who are still providing psychologically sensitive care with an outmoded theory of the brain-mind.

A Practical Guide to Neurodynamic Psychotherapy

Based on the foregoing principles, it is possible to enunciate a practical guide for the psychotherapist wishing to base his or her interventions in modern brain-mind state science while still retaining the sense of personal engagement, theoretical acuity, and depth of focus that attracted so many bright and dedicated people to psychoanalysis. In this introductory guide, I develop the set of fundamental rules that have helped me in my own transition from the psychoanalytic orientation of my training to the neurodynamic outlook of my current clinical practice.

Therapeutic Bonding: Alliance vs. Neutrality

All human beings have a strong propensity to connect actively with each other. Most patients bring to the therapeutic encounter a history of damage to this affiliation system. A prime goal of therapy is thus to identify and correct these affiliative defects. The psychoanalytic model supposes that the diagnosis and treatment of affiliative incapacity depends first upon its uncovering via free association and asserts that its reconstruction depends upon transference analysis. In order to have success with this agenda, the therapist must remain neutral, becoming a blank screen upon which the patient can project unconscious fantasies regarding, especially, problematic parents and siblings. When obstacles to the inquiry are encountered (and with doctors behaving in this peculiar way it is not surprising that they so often are encountered!), resort may be made to dreaming, the ultimate rosetta stone of the unconscious.

Contrasting with this highly artificial, abstract, and speculative approach is the actively supportive and transparently open stance of the neurodynamic psychiatrist who knows that: (1) neutrality is both unobtainable and undesirable; (2) affiliative damage is easy to perceive by direct observation; (3) affiliative damage is easy to trace by straightforward history-taking; (4) associative processes are always context dependent; (5) no association is ever truly free; (6) early memories are lost forever but can easily be fabricated in response to nonspecific demand and specific suggestions; and (7) dreams, like the histories themselves, directly reveal the fears, anger, and pain that hamper the trust and outreach needed to effect repair of affiliative deficiencies.

The construction of an alliance in psychotherapy should be an active process in which the engaged therapist takes the lead while remaining fully aware that transference is an important and self-evident aspect. With this welcoming point of view the neurodynamic psychologist begins the corrective process at once—in the first session—by offering a fully visible, corrective model of openness, comfort, and transparency. The treatment, such as it is, occurs in the here and now, through consciousness, and strives to displace the affiliative limitations with affiliative competence.

Therapeutic Process: Cooperation vs. Resistance

The investigative mission is conducted in the context of an alliance whose spirit and goals are entirely collaborative. This does away with the tension induced by the pseudo-neutrality and passivity of the Freudian psychoanalyst. Also eliminated are such concepts as resistance and regression, because neither is either necessary or helpful.

One might, in fact, see resistance as one side effect of the authoritarianism of a therapeutic model that assumes, *a priori,* that psychopathogenic mechanisms are obscure and only knowable through a process of symbol decoding by a bearded sage sitting behind us! In my experience, most patients today are only too fully aware of the adverse aspects of their affiliative training at the hands of their parents. Thanks to psychoanalysis, this information is as transparent as the emotional salience of dreams. We can thus readily make a link—without complex interpretations, without regression, and without transference—between early adversities and current dream themes.

Instead of battling against resistance to find out about the noxious affects of misguided parenting, I find myself battling against the tendency of many patients to cling to such stories as ways of justifying continuing dysfunctionality. It is this sense of the persistence of the ill effects of early life misadventure to which we might now best apply the term resistance.

Far from encouraging regression to early stages of dependency in the vain hope of reconstructing healthier affiliative behaviors, I find myself trying to prevent regression so that the patient can get on with the job of replacing the unhealthy constructs of the past with healthier ones in the present. In this connection, I do not hesitate to teach, to advocate, and even to demonstrate the active adoption of positive mental attitudes. I also encourage active approach behaviors and affiliative experimentation with whatever peers are currently available.

All of this is, of course, standard practice in cognitive behavioral therapy, and I do not pretend that it is in itself innovative. My only contribution is to show how comfortably it sits on the solid foundation of the mind-brain paradigm. At the same time, it calls forth from that paradigm a mechanistic model of change at the level of the brain, namely a shift in balance and in specific connections between the executive functions of the dorsolateral prefrontal cortex and the limbic system.

Therapeutic Model: Reconstruction vs. Catharsis

Our working assumption is that the unconscious brain-mind is fixed in some respects and plastic in others. What is fixed is the insistency of instinctual drives and the power of emotions that continue to exert their motivating and shaping forces upon affiliative behavior over the life cycle. What is plastic is the connection between instinct and emotion and the contextual contingencies in which that connection is embedded. If, from the initial encounter, affiliation is actively shaped, then its emotional associations can begin to be changed from, say, fearful and angry, to joyous and grateful even before the specific dynamics of their origins in early family life are discussed.

By placing the focus and emphasis on transparency in the here and now, therapy avoids an otherwise natural tendency to be backward looking, regressive, and resistant. The psychoanalytic assumption, deriving from the erroneous dream theory that specific psychosexual traumata must be uncovered in order to release a pathogenic complex and so liberate consciousness, is replaced by an assumption of conscious access to much more general and pervasive traumata that can be relearned by the active collusion of two people working together through consciousness to rebalance and redistribute its connections with the unconscious.

An equally important assumption is that conflict and anxiety are ubiquitous, ongoing, and recurrent not so much because of an unconscious repetitive compulsion, but rather because life is always a competitive and uncertain interaction of unknowably complex variables. In that sense, therapy is indeed "interminable" if one expects to rid the world and the brain-mind of its intrinsic chaotic properties. Rather than vainly hoping to get to the bottom of it, we should try our best to stay on top of it while fully realizing that despite our most nimble balancing efforts we will all get out of whack from time to time.

What REM sleep dreams teach us is that although nothing in the way of specific content can ever be predicted, we can be sure that our experience will always (1) be dominated by vivid sensorimotor awareness; (2) have something to do with the recent and distant past; (3) be a mix of emotions, some pleasant and some not so pleasant; (4) be accompanied by some vain attempt to make it all cohere as a strong story that we can believe and tell with confidence; and (5) we will remember some but forget most of it!

Changing Our Minds—and Bodies—for Comfort and for Health

Now that we understand how priming of the brain-mind can occur via exposure to words or visual images and how it can create an unconscious propensity to think and/or act according to the prescriptions of suggestion, we are in a stronger position to begin to answer some of the questions that have long baffled theorists and healthcare professionals. An important dimension of the processes that we will now consider is the connection of the brain-mind to and from the body. Because our model specifies participation of the brain even in transactions like hypnosis and lucid dreaming, it is easy to see how the body might be used to contribute to the desired changes of brain-mind state (e.g., muscular relaxation and eye closure). And if a change in brain-mind state is induced by any means, including purely psychological means, it follows that the body may well be its beneficiary (e.g., by saving energy, reducing blood pressure, releasing growth hormone, etc.)

The Relaxation Response

Because muscular relaxation is such a potent means of resetting brain-mind circuits and because it is an intrinsic aspect of sleep and hypnosis, it is worthwhile to begin by considering the mechanism of the relaxation response, made popular by the work of my colleague Herbert Benson, and now more easily understood and integrated by the brain-mind paradigm. Awake subjects can sense muscle tension, and then reduce it voluntarily. Reducing muscle tension has two desirable effects: it saves energy and it relieves the brain-mind of an unnecessary and unproductive allocation of valuable informational resources. Anxiety, and its cognitive companion, worry, are adaptive only up to a point beyond which the emotion takes over and gets in the way of clear thinking, emotional comfort, and effective communication. How does this work?

Keeping the muscles in a state of heightened tension prepares the body for fight or flight, but neither of these extreme reactions are usually appropriate in modern work or family settings. The minute that muscle tension begins to diminish, the whole set—or state—of the subject moves in AIM state space in the direction of sleep, but does not cross its border. In fact, relaxed waking is the way station to several other states of interest, including hypnosis, imagination, fantasy, and associative freedom. Hence the psychoanalyst's couch, hence the behaviorist's nitrous oxide, and hence the meditator's mantra.

When tense, the muscles receive strong excitatory activation from the brain and, in turn, project excitatory activation back to it. When the tension is performance anxiety—as it so often is—the positive feedback loop that perpetuates the excitatory activation of the brain and muscles include the amygdala at the expense of the dorsolateral prefrontal cortex, which is not free to work its executive functions in an adaptive way. Hence memory may be blocked, decisiveness deferred, and creativity crippled.

Anxiety and tension are thus the enemies of "flow," Czychszentmihali's wonderful term for that released condition of the mind that is both subjectively pleasant and informationally elaborative.

I hope it is clear from this discussion that the muscles can be both targets (of increased postural tone motor output) and sources (of increased sensorimotor input). They thus contribute doubly to move the input-output gating function (I) further back in the state space at the same time that the activation level (A) moves to the extreme right. The participation of the limbic system, especially the amygdala, creates a positive feedback loop that raises the level of aminergic modulation (M) toward the ceiling of the state space.

"Uptight and out of sight" is the vernacular expression for this position in state space, and "laid back," is the end result of a Californian's treatment program for uptightness. These terms nicely convey the sense of movement toward the center of AIM state space that the relaxation response enhances. Of course, it also describes the postural shift from head up, eyes focused, jaws clenched, edge of chair, and leaning forward to sitting back and looking calmly around or just gently musing to one's self.

Speaking of musing, we need to consider the role of mental content in all of this. One of the key moves of the relaxation response is to substitute natural visual imagery—a pleasant landscape, for example—for the obsessive chatter of unproductive mental noise. It's a bit like going away to the country for the weekend without getting in to your car. Here again, as in hypnosis and lucid dreaming, one makes a voluntary decision to prime the brain-mind and so change its focus, its rate of production, and its subject matter by means of simple autosuggestion. In this case, however, we are not counting on an unconscious incubation that will later emerge in another state so much as we are directly and immediately preempting working memory to get it out of the perseveration mode. Once we have created an interrupt and forced the mind from the obsession with irrelevant details, we can use it to accomplish a variety of other purposes, from the existential satisfaction of just being to the search for innovative solutions to intellectual problems.

If we are successful in reducing the output of high levels of excitatory drive to the muscles, and if we can interrupt the positive feedback loop that activates the amygdala, then the sympathetic outflow as well as the somatic outflow will decline. As a consequence our heart rate will fall, our respiration will deepen and slow, our blood pressure will decline, and in time, our adrenocortical hormone release will go down.

This link of central state to peripheral outflow unifies Hans Selye's concept of stress to Cannon's fight or flight paradigm and places both in a model that specifies, to a first approximation, the way that brain-mind state control systems can coordinate the complex array of processes that are involved. The twin beneficiaries of our model and the interventions illuminated by it are nothing less than mental and bodily health.

Transcendental Meditation

The goals of transcendental meditation are similar to those of the relaxation response. Being derived from Eastern mystical practices, they have a distinctive philosophical and cultural spin. Instead of seeking to instill identifiable and tranquilizing mental content, transcendental meditation practitioners seek a state of consciousness that is devoid of content. This contentless consciousness is believed to be pre- or extra-existential, cosmic, or otherworldly; hence the term "transcendental." It is this reconnection with primordial, universal, preverbal awareness that confers the benefit of transcendental meditation. Here we are clearly in religious territory.

Without wishing to challenge the belief systems of transcendental meditation adepts, it is possible to propose a mechanistic explanation along the same lines as those used to analyze hypnotic phenomena and lucid dreaming. In the case of transcendental meditation, the subject wishes to remain awake—or at least remain aware—but to be free of directed thoughts, organized precepts, and internal language.

The key to understanding the difference between transcendental meditation and its altered state first cousins—hypnosis and lucid dreaming—is the use of the mantra in the autosuggestion induction routine. The mantra is a semi-verbal prime. It seeks to occupy working memory networks of the dorsolateral prefrontal cortex with a subcognitive program whose meaning is metaphysically linked to the state of reunification the practitioner seeks. Each practitioner is encouraged to find his or her own mantra, the more primitive and nonverbal the better. Hence the epigrammatic OM! of the Buddhists.

On hearing the OM! and while focusing my mind on my increasingly deep and slow breathing, I drop down and out of the verbal world into a sea of pure color or pure colorlessness or pure sound or pure silence. It's nice. It's soft. It's warm. I'm reconnected to source. By using a mantra I also avoid the trap of trying *not* to think of elephants, alligators, the stock market, or my mother-in-law.

Come to think of it, the use of OM! may move my brain-mind closer to the musical domain, where music is defined as a preverbal and pre-programmatic sequence of sounds. When I listen to music, especially impressionistic music by Debussy or Ravel, I can sometimes enter a transcendental meditation-like state of consciousness that is pleasurably nonanalytic. But it's hard, because I am always in danger of either rising up to my usual state of verbal rumination or of falling through the floor of relaxed, off-line waking, into the black hole of sleep (especially if I am sleep deprived and the concert is in the evening, as it so often is!).

Just as some of us were never destined for trance, so some of us were not cut out for transcendence. What this means is that the zones of the state space that we can or can't enter are more or less accessible on an individual basis. And that individual basis—like long and short sleep, high and low energy, logical and analogical cognition—is both genetic-constitutional-trait bound, as well as environmental-cultural-state determined.

Individual Differences and the Power of Positive Thinking

To understand the brain basis of individuality as it pertains to hypnotiz-ability, lucidity, relaxation, and transcendental meditation, it is helpful to recognize as a didactic example how early in life traits like extroversion and introversion appear and how indelibly they persist. The child who at age five is outgoing, unselfconscious, and socially gregarious is father of the man who at age fifty is enthusiastically involved in a multiplicity of work and social projects, whereas the child who is fearful and timid is likely later in life to prefer narrow and clearly defined vocational and social roles, often pursued alone.

The bridge from dispositional affect to the topics of our interest comes via still another striking example of regional activation differences in the brain. The reader will probably not be surprised to learn that this regional difference involves the frontal cortex, but this time on a side-to-side rather than top-to-bottom basis. People who are optimistic, socially engaged, and outgoing tend to have greater levels of brain activation in their left frontal lobes, whereas their more doubtful, private, and reserved fellows have greater levels of brain activation in their right frontal lobes!

This lateralization difference is measurable using EEG technology, which puts it on more solid ground than the seductive but related idea that the left brain is the logical verbal organizer and the right brain is the parallel, intuitive, emotional feeler in all of us. We don't yet know the degree to which these traits correlate with the optimism-pessimism dichotomy and we don't know whether left or right frontal dominance is more hypnotizable, lucid, or relaxation prone, but we can at least be sure that, like handedness, whatever clusters emerge are likely to be set early in life.

The upshot of this—for an optimist like me at least—is not despair at my genetically imposed limitations. It is rather the conscious affirmation of those patterns that are easy for me to follow and philosophical acceptance of those that are difficult. So what if I am not trance or transcendence bound? I can still use auto-suggestion to achieve enough anesthesia to tolerate my dentist and enough dream lucidity to convince myself of its veracity and enjoy its pleasures. Why should I beat my head against the built-in barriers of my own AIM state space? Why not go with the flow, in my case along the inviting path of linear logical thought with enough openness to emotion and associativity to do psychotherapy, write books, and have a deeply satisfying love life!

The new phrenology of the state space era is thus a three-dimensional map of each individual's predisposition to occupy the several domains of AIM and of each individual's capacity to move in and out of those hinterland domains that confer pleasure or enlightenment. It goes without saying that a corollary benefit is the characterization of our predilection for the risks of pathological excess, including those of mental illness, and of possibly adverse response to drugs.

Bibliography

Barger, F. M. The use of antianxiety drugs. *Clinical Pharmacology and Therapeutics* 29:291, 1981.

De Quincey, Thomas. *Confessions of an English Opium-Eater.* New York: Dover Publications, Inc., 1995.

Grinspoon, Lester, and Bakalar, James B. *Psychedelic Drugs Reconsidered.* New York: The Lindesmith Center, 1997.

Grinspoon, Lester, and Bakalar, James B. (eds.). *Psychedelic Reflections.* New York: Human Sciences Press, Inc., 1983.

Hobson, J. Allan. *The Dreaming Brain.* New York: Basic Books, 1988.

Hobson, J. Allan. *Sleep.* New York: Scientific American Library, 1989.

Hobson, J. Allan. *Consciousness.* New York: Scientific American Library, 1989.

Hobson, J. Allan. Sleep and dreaming. In M. J. Zigmond and F. E. Bloom (eds.), *Fundamental Neuroscience.* New York: Academic Press, 1998.

Hobson, J. Allan. *Dreaming as Delirium.* Cambridge: MIT Press, 1999.

Hofmann, Albert. *LSD: My Problem Child.* New York: McGraw-Hill Book Co., 1980.

Klüver, Heinrich. *Mescal and Mechanisms of Hallucinations.* Chicago: The University of Chicago Press, 1966.

Schultes, Richard Evans, and Hofmann, Albert. *Plants of the Gods.* Rochester, VT: Healing Arts Press, 1992.

Snyder, Solomon H. *Drugs and the Brain.* New York: Scientific American Books, Inc., 1986.

Solms, Mark. *The Neuropsychology of Dreams.* Mahwah, NJ: Lawrence Erlbaum Associates, Inc., 1997.

Tart, Charles T. (ed.). *Altered States of Consciousness: A Book of Readings.* New York: John Wiley & Sons, Inc. 1969.

Index

Dreams (cont.)
  physiological differences between
    waking and, 57
  priming, 31–35, 96–97
  vs. psychedelic drug states, 284–285
  and psychoanalysis, 70–71
  psychosis, 231–232, 240, 259
  and psychotherapy, 79–82
  and REM sleep, 50–53
  and selective serotonin receptor in-
    hibitors (SSRIs), 43
  and self-hypnosis, 94–96
  and sensation, 260–261
  and serotonin, 257–258
  sleep onset, 155–156
  spontaneity in, 29–30
  and stroke, 181–187
  and supramarginal gyrus, 185–187,
    193–194
  and temporal lobe epilepsy (TLE),
    197
  and thalamocortical system, 178
  and trances, 109
  and visual imagery, 73–74, 295–298
  and waking consciousness, 49–66
  as wish fulfillments, 190–191
Drugs. See also Amphetamines; Bar-
    biturates; Cocaine; LSD; Mesca-
    line; Opium
  action on the waking brain, 35–42
  administration timing, 207–209
  antidepressant, 219–229
  antiepileptic, 244–247
  antipsychotic, 210, 234–235, 236–
    237
  benzodiazepines, 214–218
  clean and dirty, 211–214
  habitual use of, 150
  half-life of, 209–211
  localization of action of, 206–207
  monoamine oxidase inhibitors, 220–
    221, 223
  and narcolepsy, 169
  phencyclidine (PCP), 241–244
  from plants, 287–303
  psychedelic
    action on the brain, 35–42

  and the cult of dreaming, 294–298
  discovery of, 25–26
  vs. dreams, 284–285
  and mental illness, 38, 43–44
  in psychotherapy, 82–84
  psychotogenic, 251–252
    biochemistry of, 267–269
    and central aminergic demodula-
      tion, 265–267
    and serotonin, 267–269
    and serotonin-dopamine interaction,
      26
  stimulant, 235–236
  and tardive dyskinesia, 209–210
  Thorazine, 24–25, 26, 228–229
  and tranquilization, 24–25
Dualism, 18

Ecstasy, 4, 149, 288
Electroencephalograms (EEGs), 49, 51
  and brain internal pulse generator in
    REM sleep, 139–142
Electromyograms (EMGs), 50
Electrooculograms (EOGs), 50
Eltoprazine, 43
Emotional salience, 10, 53, 59–61,
    71–72
Emotions. See also Anxiety; Depres-
    sion
  aggression, 261
  anger, 78, 196, 293
  and dreaming, 261
  elation, 261, 274–275
  fear, 155, 196, 261, 275–276, 293
  and forebrain activation model of
    dreaming, 188–190
  and heroin, 274–275
  and LSD, 258–259
  mania, 77, 196, 232, 244–247
  and mescaline, 293
  and morphine, 274–275
  and temporal lobe epilepsy (TLE),
    196
Endogenous analgesia, 273–276
Endorphins, 274
Enkephalins, 274
Environmental insult, 238

Printed in the United States
by Baker & Taylor Publisher Services